Keto Breakfast Cookbook

Easy Meal Prep Recipes for High Protein Low Carbs Breakfast

By

Adele Tyler

The trademarks that are used are without any consent, and the publication of the trademark is without permission or backing by the trademark owner. All trademarks and brands within this book are for clarifying purposes only and are the owned by the owners themselves, not affiliated with this document.

Table Of Contents

CHAPTER 5: SWEET RECIPES FOR KETO BREAKFAST..91

Introduction

Ketogenic is a term for a low-carb diet (like the Atkins diet). The idea is for you to get more calories from protein and fat and less from carbohydrates. You cut back most on the carbs that are easy to digest, like sugar, soda, pastries, and white bread. When you eat less than 50 grams of carbs a day, your body eventually runs out of fuel, and it is used quickly. This typically takes 3 to 4 days. Then you'll start to break down protein and fat for energy, which can make you lose weight. This is called ketosis. It's important to note that the ketogenic diet is a short-term diet that's focused on weight loss rather than the pursuit of health benefits. People simply use a ketogenic diet most often to lose weight, but it can help manage certain medical conditions, like epilepsy, too. It also may help people with heart disease, certain brain diseases, and even acne, but there needs to be more. Because there's such a high-fat necessity in the keto diet, followers must eat fat at each meal. That might look like 165 grams of fat, 40 grams of carbs, and 75 grams of protein in a daily 2,000-calorie diet. The exact ratio, however, depends on your specific needs.

Keto diet allows for some healthy unsaturated fats — like nuts (walnuts, almonds), seeds, tofu, avocados, and olive oil. Yet large levels of saturated fats are recommended from oils (coconut, palm), butter, lard, and cocoa butter. Protein is a major component of the keto diet but typically does not differentiate between lean protein food and protein sources rich in saturated fat like beef, bacon, and pork. What about Vegetables and Fruits? All fruits are high in carbs, but in small portions, you can get specific fruits (generally berries)Vegetables (also high in carbs) are confined to leafy greens (including kale, chard, Swiss, spinach), broccoli, cauliflower, brussels sprouts, bell peppers, asparagus, tomatoes, garlic, mushrooms, cucumbers, summer squashes, and celery. A cup of broccoli is chopped and has almost six carbs. While it also has some potential keto risks as well, including liver deficiency, liver-related issues, constipation, kidney problems, etc. So, we should balance our Keto diet amounts too.

Chapter 1: Understanding the Fundamentals of the Ketogenic Diet

This chapter gives detail about the Ketogenic diet. Which foods to eat under the Keto diet and which foods to avoid while having this diet also includes in the chapter. The way keto diet works and what are the health benefits are also discussed in detail and depth.

The ketogenic diet (or, in short, keto diet) is a high-fat, low carb diet that has many health-related benefits. Indeed, more than twenty studies indicate that this type of diet can help you to improve your health and lose weight. Ketogenic diets could even benefit from diabetes, epilepsy, Alzheimer's disease, and cancer.

1.1 What is Keto?

The ketogenic diet consists of a low-carb diet with a high-fat content that shares many familiarities with the Atkins diets and diets, which are low-carb. It requires a dramatic decrease in the use of carbohydrates and the substitution with fat. This decrease in carbs places your body in a metabolic state, which is called ketosis. Whenever this happens, the body becomes extremely efficient in energy in burning fat. And it also transforms fat into the form ketones in your liver that can provide the brain with the energy. Keto diets can lead to massive decreases in insulin levels and blood sugar. This, with the heightened ketones, that has many health benefits.

Varieties of Ketogenic Diets:

Few versions of the ketogenic diet exist including:

The standard ketogenic diet: A diet that is extremely low in carbohydrates, moderate in protein, as well as high in fats. It typically contains 75% fat, just 5% carbs, and 20% protein.

The cyclic ketogenic diet: That is, the diet involves high-carb reefed periods, such as five ketogenic days being followed by two high-carbohydrate days.

A targeted ketogenic diet: The diet enables carbs to be added around the workouts.

Protein-rich ketogenic diet: This is close to a regular keto diet, except more protein is used. The proportion is often 60% fat, 5% carbs, and 35% protein.

However, as there has been extensive study only on standard and protein high ketogenic diets. Targeted or cyclic keto diets are more advanced methods and are used primarily by bodybuilders and athletes.

Health benefits of Ketogenic Diet:

In reality, the keto diet emerged as a method for treating disorders, which are neurological, including disease named epilepsy. Next, studies have demonstrated that diet can benefit a wide range of various conditions of health:

Diseases of heart: The keto diet may improve risk-related factors such as levels of HDL cholesterol, body fat, blood sugar, and blood pressure.

Alzheimer's disease: The ketogenic diet will reduce Alzheimer's disease symptoms and also delay further development.

- **Epilepsy**

Research has shown us that diet named as ketogenic diet in children with epileptic seizures can cause massive decreases in seizures.

- **Cancer**

The diet is used to treat multiple cancer types and slow growth of the tumors.

- **Acne**

Reduced rates of insulin also fewer intakes of sugar or fried products will help to boost acne treatment.

- **Parkinson's Disease**

One study found that diet also had helped improve Parkinson's disease symptoms.

- **Brain Injuries**

One test showed the diet is capable of increasing concussions as well as improving healing following brain injury.

- **Polycystic Ovary Syndrome**

Ketogenic diet can aid reduce insulin rates and may play a crucial role in the condition of polycystic ovary.

Foods you can eat under Ketogenic Diet:

Most of your meals will be centered on certain foods:

- **Fatty Fish**

Salmon, mackerel, trout, and tuna, for example.

- **Eggs**

Look for whole eggs, pastured, or omega-3.

- **Butter and Cream**

When possible, look for grass-fed.

- **Meat**

Red meat, sausage, ham, turkey, chicken, bacon, and steak.

- **Cheese**

Cheese (cheddar, goat, mozzarella, blue, or cream) not processed.

- **Nuts and Beans**

Seeds from flax, pumpkin seeds, walnuts, seeds from chia, almonds, etc.

- **Healthy Oils**

Mainly avocado oil, coconut oil, and extra virgin olive oil.

- **Condiments**

Salt, pepper, and spices, and various healthy herbs can be used.

- **Avocados**

Complete avocados or freshly produced guacamole.

- **Low-Carb Vegetables**

Certain green veggies, tomatoes, peppers, onions, and so on.

The best way to base your diet on the whole, single-ingredient foods is it.

Foods you should avoid under Ketogenic Diet:

Any food that is carb-rich should be kept to a minimum.

A list of foods which a keto diet requires to minimize or eliminate:

- **Sugary Foods**

Fruit juice, ice cream, smoothies, soda, candy, cake, etc.

- **Starches or Grains**

Products made from wheat, cereals, pasta, rice, etc.

- **Tubers and Root Vegetables**

Sweet potatoes, parsnips, carrots, potatoes, etc.

- **Items of Reduced-Diet or Fat**

They are heavily refined and also rich in carbohydrates.

- **Fruit**

All of the fruits, excluding tiny parts of berries such as strawberries.

- **Legumes or Beans**

Chickpeas, peas, lentils, kidney beans, etc.

- **Few Sauces or Condiments**

Unhealthy fat and sugar are often present in these.

- **Fats that are Unhealthy**

Restrict your consumption of mayonnaise, refined vegetable oils, etc.

- **Alcohol**

Many alcoholic drinks can bring you off ketosis because of their carb material.

- **Sugar-Free Dietary Foods**

Mostly high in sugar amounts are alcohol that, in some cases, may affect the ketone levels. These products seem to be refined extensively, too.

Some basic foods to eat while being on a Ketogenic diet:

Low-Carb Vegetables:

Starch fewer veggies are low regarding carbs and calories, but also high in numerous nutrients, having a few minerals and vitamin C. Vegetables, as well as other plants, produce fiber that is not digested and consumed by the body like other carbohydrates.

Consider their digestible count of carb, which would be the total carbohydrates while minus fiber. Most of the veggies contain a lot of carbs, which are net. Nevertheless, consuming a single serving of those vegetables having starch such as beets or yams, potatoes, could make you on your entire daytime carb limit. Among non-starchy foods, the net count of carb changes from may less than one gram among one cup of uncooked spinach to eight grams for one cup of Brussels sprouts, which are cooked. There are also antioxidants in vegetables that help guard against the free radicals that are not stable molecules that can kill cells. Moreover, cruciferous veggies such as broccoli, cauliflower, and kale, have been associated with a reduced risk of heart disease and cancer. Low-carb vegetables are developing excellent replacements for carb products, which are high. Cauliflower, for starters, can be used either to replicate mashed potatoes or rice, noodles that can be formed from spaghetti squash and zucchini is the best substitute for spaghetti.

Avocados:

Avocados are fantastically healthy. 3.5 ounces, or almost half of a medium-sized avocado, produce 9 grams of carbs. Seven of these are fiber, however, so its net carb number is just 2 of grams. Avocados are high in few minerals and vitamins, including potassium. Many individuals might not get enough of this important mineral. What's more, an increased intake of potassium may help facilitate the transition towards a keto diet. Additionally, avocados can help boost triglyceride levels and cholesterol. In a study, they experienced a 22 percent decline in "bad" triglycerides and LDL cholesterol while an 11 percent increase in "good "cholesterol named HDL when people used a diet that is high in avocados.

Seafood:

Shellfish and fish are products that are really pleasant to the keto. Some fishes and Salmon are very rich in vitamins B, selenium, and potassium but are virtually free from carbon. The carbs differ in different forms of shellfish, however. For example, while the most crabs and shrimp do not contain carbs, other shellfish types have. While these shellfish can be involved in a keto diet, when you are trying to stay within a small range, it's significant to account for all these carbs. Here are the carb counts of some common shellfish forms for 3.5-ounce servings:

Clams: 5 grams

Oysters: 4 grams

Octopus: 4 grams

Squid: 3 grams

Mussels: 7 grams.

Salmon, mackerel, other fatty fish and sardines, are very rich in fats named omega-3, which have been shown to reduce insulin rates and improve overweight and obese people's vulnerability to insulin. Additionally, daily consumption of fish has been correlated with decreased disease risk and enhanced mental wellbeing. Aim to utilize at least two servings of seafood each week.

Cheese:

The cheese is equally savory and tasty. There are many various forms of cheese. Luckily these are all high in fat, and in carbs, they are very low, making them a perfect fit for a keto diet. A single ounce of cheddar named cheese (28 grams) provides seven grams of protein, one gram of carbs, and 20 percent of calcium RDI. Cheese is rich in saturated fat, but the incidence of heart failure hasn't been shown to rise. In fact, some studies suggest cheese can help prevent diseases of the heart. Cheese also includes a conjugated form of linoleic acid, which is a fat that has been associated with fat loss and body composition improvements. Additionally, eating your cheese regularly can help to reduce muscle mass loss and agility that happens with aging. 12-week research of older adults showed that who were eating 7 ounces of cheese named ricotta a day reported improvements of muscle power and muscle mass during the period.

Eggs:

An egg is among the planet's healthful and the flexible proteins. A big egg comprises fewer than six grams of nutrient protein as well as less than one gram of carbohydrates, rendering the eggs a perfect keto lifestyle meal. Additionally, the eggs that have been observed to activate the hormones which improve fullness feelings and regulate blood sugar rates, contributing to reduced intakes of calorie for time up to a total of 24 hours. Eating the complete egg is important since most of the nutrients of an egg are figured in the egg yolk. This involves the zeaxanthin and lutein antioxidants, which help to protect the health of the eyes. Although yolks of eggs are high in levels of cholesterol, in most individuals, utilizing these does not elevate your blood containing levels of cholesterol. In reality, eggs tend to make changes in the LDL type in such a way that decreases cardiovascular disease risk.

Cottage cheese and simple Greek yogurt:

Cottage cheese and simple Greek yogurt are healthy foods that are high in protein. They may still be included with the ketogenic lifestyle, although they consist of some carbs. Five ounces of simple Greek yogurt (150 grams) yield eleven grams of protein and five grams of carbs. That cottage cheese supplies eighteen grams protein and five grams of carbs. It has been shown that both cottage cheese and yogurt help to promote feelings of wholeness and lower your appetite. You make your own savory snack, either. But for an easy and quick keto treat, both can also be integrated with chopped nuts, optional sugar-free sweetener, and cinnamon.

Cream and Butter:

Cream and butter are healthful fats for transitioning into a keto diet. Each one only includes minor amounts of per serving carbs. Cream and butter were considered to contribute or cause heart disease for many years because of their high content of saturated fat. Several large studies, however, have shown that saturated fat is not associated with heart disease for most people. In reality, some studies suggested that moderate high dairy fat consumption could potentially reduce the danger of stroke and heart attack. Butter and cream, like the other fatty milk products, which are highly rich in fatty acids that can promote loss of fat and conjugated linoleic acid.

Olives:

Olives, even in strong shape, offer similar health-related benefits of olive oil. The major antioxidant, which is discovered in olives, Oleuropein has against-inflammatory characteristics and can protect the cells against damage. Furthermore, research shows that olive intake can help avoid rising blood pressure and bone loss. Due to the size, the olives differ in carb quality. Half of the carbohydrates, though, emerge from fiber, and they have a very poor digestible quality of carb. A single ounce olive serving provides 1 gram of fiber and two grams of net carbs. Based on their height, this works against the net carb amount of one gram for 8–10 olives.

1.2 How the Keto diet works?

The "ketogenic" keto diet includes eating a middle amount of protein, a high amount of fat, and very fewer carbs, even fruit is off from the table. As with any diet fad, followers all of the benefits include increased energy, weight loss, and increased cognitive clarity. But is the ketogenic diet all cracked up for it to be?

Dietitians and nutritionists are not exactly saying. Low-carb diets such as keto also tend to contribute to any weight reduction in the short term, but they are not substantially greater success than any other self-help or mainstream diet. And they do not seem to be improving sports performance.

The ketogenic diet was initially formulated for epilepsy rather than weight reduction. Doctors discovered in the 1920s that maintaining the patients on diets which are low in carbs caused their bodies to consume fat as the very first-line fuel supply, rather than the normal glucose. The body changes the fats into the fatty acids when only fat is accessible for the body to combust or burn and then into the compounds called ketones that can be used and taken up to fuel the cells of the body.

Still now, feeding the body on main ketones decreases seizures for purposes not entirely known. However, few patients with epilepsy depend on ketogenic diets nowadays with the advancement of the drugs, which are anti-seizure, although certain individuals who may not react to medicines may also gain. For weight reduction, keto diets today are the products of low carb diets such as the Atkins diet, that rose in prominence in the early 2000s. And both forms of diets in favor of meatier meals avoid carbohydrates. The keto diet does not have a clear outline, but schedules typically allow for consuming less than fifty grams of carbs a day.

A keto diet drives the body into a condition called ketosis, which implies that the cells of the body become essentially dependent on ketones for the energy. Why that contributes to weight loss is not completely obvious, but ketosis tends to reduce hunger and may influence hormones such as insulin that control hunger. Proteins and fats will, therefore, hold humans fuller as compared to carbohydrates, contributing to lower average calorie consumption.

Researchers examined 48 distinct diet experiments in one head-to-head comparison, in which respondents were assigned randomly to one of several famous diets. The diets included low-carb diets such as South Beach, Atkins, and Zone, as well as low-fat containing diets such as Ornish diets, and portion control diets such as Weight Watchers and Jenny Craig.

There observed that after six months, every diet culminated in greater weight loss than almost no diet. L ow-carb and low-fat diets were practically identical, with dieters of low-carb losing

19 pounds (8.73 kilograms) on average and low-fat dieters losing 17.6 pounds (7.99 kg) on average, as relative to non-dieters. The effects demonstrated signs of a falling off for all diet forms at 12 months, with low-fat and low-carb dieters showing 16 pounds (7.27 kg) thinner on average than non-dieters.

Differences in weight loss between named person diets were low. This follows the tradition of suggesting every diet an individual adheres to with a view to reducing weight.

Another analysis of famous diets discovered the Atkins diet that results in more reduction of weight than simply educating individuals on portion control, but also recognized that most of the research papers of this low-carb diet involved authorized dietitians helping respondents make food choices, instead of the self-directed procedure by which most individuals take the diets. That's true in other diet experiments, the researchers noted, and the findings of the analysis actually seem rosier in the actual world than the weight loss.

Finally, a straightforward analysis between low-carb and low-fat dieting showed that there was a little statistically meaningful disparity in the figure of weight reduced over a year. The low-carbohydrate dieters shed an average of 13 pounds (6 kg), while low-fat dieters lost a total of 11.7 pounds (5.3 kg).

Ketogenic diets can help us reduce weight, but they are no more helpful compared to other strategies of diet. Since carbohydrate stocks in the body hold molecules of water with them, most of the weight removed in the early phases of a ketogenic diet is water weight. This initially pushes the scale a thrilling number, but weight loss eventually slows over time.

Keto benefits; how it helps?

A keto diet has similar benefits to those other higher-fat and low-carb diets, but it seems more potent than centrist low-carb diets. Find keto as a low-carb, super-charged diet that maximizes the benefits. It can also boost the risk of complications a little bit, however.

Help to lose weight:

Turning the body into a fat-burning system will improve weight loss. Fat burning is increased significantly, while insulin levels – the hormone that stores fat – are dropping sharply. This appears to make it much simpler for loss of body fat to arise, without starvation.

More than Thirty high-quality clinical reports indicate that low-carb and keto diets provide a more efficient weight reduction relative to other diets.

Control Blood Sugar

Research shows that a ketogenic diet is outstanding for the management of type 2 diabetes, occasionally leading even to complete disease reversal. It makes complete sense, as keto eliminates the need for treatment, decreases levels of blood sugar, and eliminates the possible adverse effects of elevated levels of insulin.

Since a keto diet can overturn existing type 2 diabetes, prevention and reversal of pre-diabetes are likely to be effective. Remember that in this sense, the word "reversal" actually implies improving the condition, increasing glucose regulation, and reducing the need for treatment. At all, it can be so much changed that without treatment, blood pressure falls to usual, long-term. In this sense, reversal means moving ahead or getting worse in the opposite direction of the disease. Lifestyle changes, though, just work if you do them. If an individual returns to the style of living he or she experienced when diabetes type 2 appeared and progressed, it is likely to come back and get success again over time.

Boost up energy and mental performance:

Some people actually use ketogenic diets for better mental output. Also, when in ketosis, it is common for individuals to experience a boost in energy.

On keto, they don't require dietary carbohydrates for the brain. It's fueled by ketones 24-7 coupled with a limited volume of synthesized glucose from the liver. Dietary carbohydrates are not required. Hence, ketosis contributes to a constant supply of fuel (ketones) towards the brain, thereby preventing issues with major fluctuations of blood sugar. This can also contribute to increased attention and concentrate, and brain fog clearance, with enhanced mental clarity.

Treats Epilepsy:

The keto diet is an established, and still successful, epileptic medical treatment used since 19 and 20s. It has traditionally been used particularly for children, but it has also benefited adults in recent years. Using a keto diet for epilepsy may enable some individuals to take less or none of the anti-epileptic medications while staying potentially seizure-free. This may reduce the side effects of the drug and thus enhance cognitive performance.

Chapter 2: Importance of Breakfast and Daily Keto Routine

Your dietary prescription is designed around your specific nutritional requirements, based on your activity level, your normal diet, and any nutrient deficiencies that may have emerged from your baseline screening. Meals and snacks are based on a simple combination of foods that are rich in a wide range of nutrients. You are encouraged to choose as much variety of foods as possible.

2.1 Why Breakfast is Important in the Ketogenic Diet?

Taking a nutritious breakfast is in decline for both adults and babies. Between teens, the pattern is much more prominent. The root cause? A hectic and stressful life decreased in the morning, with time devoted to breakfast. It's clear this meal is often ignored. It is a gentle reminder that breakfast is vital to our reasoning skills, our wellbeing, our weight. Starved by ten to twelve hours of overnight fasting, our body has a critical need to refuel its morning battery. Actually, that's where its name comes from, breaking the fast! A healthy breakfast aims to supply our bodies with certain important nutrients: proteins, minerals, micro-nutrients, vitamins, fibers. There is a desire to relieve our appetite with high sugar and unhealthy snacks at mid-morning, in the absence of breakfast. There should be a good breakfast, including:

- A beer, at least one-quarter liter. The bodies have worked vigorously at night to remove the urine. We become dehydrated in the morning, without even noticing it. Such exhaustion may then be the cause of specific muscle fatigue if it is not completed. Milk can be a good breakfast companion if it mixes sugar, calcium, and protein. Unless the child may not want milk, substitute it with a fruit pulp drink, and calcium that be offered as dairy products. Are you hooked to coffee?

- Cereals: they can add nutrition to the rest of the morning, high in sugars and carbohydrates; Focus on honey toast, jelly, and butter, or margarine, consider mixing.

- Proteins contained in dairy foods, poultry, eggs (try to locate organic eggs, because they have more omega3 than regular eggs) or nuts. We offer the sensation of being full faster and longer and are important for proper muscle and brain functioning.

- Great sources of vitamins and minerals are fruit and vegetables, so aim to have a part of your regular five at breakfast.

So don't forget to take your time, sit down, and have a good meal. Prepare for 5 minutes, feed for 10 minutes. This would be the day's biggest purchase, and you will bring three bonus advantages to the meal: gustatory satisfaction, comfort, and conviviality.

2.2 Preparing your Breakfast According to Your Macros

Carbohydrate containing foods; a significant reduction

Carbohydrate control is fundamental to the ketogenic fuel switch, and a therapeutic ketogenic diet for adults will generally contain 20-30g carbohydrates per day. I recommend choosing carbohydrate-containing foods that release their glucose more slowly, such as non-starchy vegetables, berries, dairy products, nuts, and seeds, to provide your prescribed amounts at meals. Weight for weight, these foods are also much lower in carbohydrate than traditional starchy sources, so you can get more food bulk for your carbohydrate allowance. On ketogenic diets, whenever any carbohydrate is eaten, there always needs to be some fat alongside this.

Fats and oils; a significant change from 'normal.'

Fats are the main driver for ketone production and become your main fuel, needing to be included in each meal and snack. Examples of good fat sources are olive oil, coconut oil, butter, lard, double cream, mayonnaise, avocados, nuts, and cheese. Protein containing foods such as meats, oily fish, and eggs in your meals do naturally provide some fats too, but the amounts are not adequate, so extra pure fats need to be added at each meal.

Protein containing foods; 'normal' quantities based on appetite

You will be encouraged to include a normal-sized portion of meat or fish or eggs or nuts or cheese with each meal. On a Modified ketogenic diet, protein foods are not weighed and measured, but large portions can deliver much more protein than your body needs, with the excess being burned for fuel. This reduces the need for your body to burn as much fat, impairing ketone production.

Vitamin, mineral and micronutrient supplements

Baseline vitamin, mineral, and trace element supplementation are generally recommended alongside ketogenic therapy. This can be provided by a good quality one-a-day A-Z type product aimed at adults. However, very few of these provide calcium, magnesium, and Vitamin D in adequate amounts; therefore, an additional product may be required.

Chapter 3: Different Keto Breakfast Recipe

This chapter will aid you to learn and experiment with the different basic varieties of recipes that are consumed daily in the breakfast timing or as starters regarding the Ketogenic diet. It definitely consists of an infinite number of options to try according to your flavor.

3.1 Fluffy Coconut Pancakes

You'll enjoy these pancakes with light and crispy coconut flour. This is an easy, sugar-free, and low carb recipe.

Cuisine: British, Course: Breakfast, Prep Time: 5 minutes, Cook Time: 5 minutes, Total Time: 10 minutes, Calories: 204kcal, Servings: 6 pancakes

Ingredients:

- 1 tsp. Lakanto maple-flavored syrup or sweetener of choice (optional)
- 4 tablespoon coconut flour
- 1 tbsp almond milk or coconut milk
- 1/2 cup butter/coconut oil melted (90g)
- 1 teaspoon baking powder
- 1 tsp mixed spice or pumpkin spice (you can also use cinnamon)
- 4 eggs

Instructions:

Melt butter/coconut oil then, if necessary, blend along with the coconut flour, egg yolks, coconut milk, and baking powder, then spice/sweetener. You can achieve this using a processor of food, so you should always use a blender named stick blender. If you are using a fork, first sift your coconut flour, so it doesn't stack and use a little elbow grease to have the mixture smooth and nice.

Whisk the egg whites in a bowl of porcelain or metal, until a little hard peaks form. As the stiffer, you have the whites, softer the pancakes sound.

Pull the whites of the egg into the mix.

Steam some butter in a non-stick oven, or coconut oil. This combination allows 6 pancakes (each about 10 cm in diameter) using 3 tablespoons of batter for each pancake. Then fry them over low flame medium heat to prevent them from frying. Flip over until the rim starts to bubble.

Recipe Notes:

The filled pancakes-this is the essence of coconut flour. You will want to measure two per adult if you have a hungry husband, an adult, or a busy day ahead of you. You know our persons best and the sums rise accordingly.

Nutrition:

Calories: 204kcal | Protein: 5.1g | Fiber: 2.1g | Fat: 18.9g | Carbohydrates: 3.7g | Saturated Fat: 14.3g | Monounsaturated Fat: 2.1g | Cholesterol: 124mg | Polyunsaturated Fat: 0.9g |Sodium: 60mg | Potassium: 49mg | Sugar: 0.7g

3.2 Keto Bagels Recipe (low carb)

An easy recipe for keto bagels with dough named fathead that results in amazing keto bagels at any time. Have the bagels ready for your upcoming lunch or breakfast in minutes.

Servings: 6, Cuisine: American, Prep Time: 10 minutes, Course: Breakfast, Cook Time: 12 minutes, Total Time: 22 minutes, Calories: 245kcal

Ingredients:

- 1 tbsp baking powder

- Two ounces full-fat cream cheese, cut into pieces

- 1 1/2 cup part-skim shredded mozzarella cheese (about 6 ounces)

- 1 1/4 cup almond flour

- 1 large egg

- 1 tbsp oat fiber (or you can also take 2 tbsp whey protein powder or 1/4th cup almond flour)

Directions:

You have to place the cream cheese and mozzarella in a microwave and a microwave-safe pot for one minute. Then stir and microwave for a full 30 seconds to a minute. Scrape your cheese with an egg into an eating processor and cycle until smooth.

Attach the dry ingredients then start processing until dough develops. It's getting really hot. Scrape on a sheet of fastening film and placed it in the freezer.

Heat the oven to 400 F and then place the rack in the oven center. Top a parchment-filled baking dish.

Remove your dough of bagels from your freezer when the oven is ready, and divide it into equal six pieces. Hands lightly oil and roll every part into a shape of a snake, sealing the ends all together to form a ring. Then place on the baking parchment and top up with favorite overlay, gently pressing to attach.

Bake for about twelve minutes, or you can bake until browning on the surface. They would still be fluffy, and let them cool off from your baking sheet before removing. When cold, lock in the fridge in a jar. Warm-up somewhat to toast or enjoy.

Then makes six bagels average in size. By dividing your dough into eight pieces, results in small bagels and by dividing bagels of gourmet sized into 4 results.

Keep the bagels in a container that is airtight in the refrigerator. They keep and freeze well for 7-10 days.

It is a recipe of low carb that doesn't have a real bagel's chew. They are, however, a great replacement for those who skip food.

The fiber choice for oats tastes very yummy, but use what you've got. There is comparatively biscuity to the form. If you decide on that route, your protein powder form gives an intense smooth texture.

Start inserting 2 tablespoons or 1/4 cups further almond flour as the bagels flatten out when baking. Try the trick of the baker preheating a pan of metal in the lower side of your oven and throwing cubes of ice into it when your bagels go in the oven. Then the steam will push the bagels upwards. Don't take the bagels off the pan until they get cool down a little bit.

And if your dough after mixing is lukewarm to touch, you do not need to place it into the refrigerator to cool down.

Do not repeat the formula when it's produced in the blender, or it will go under the rim. Mine had a hard time washing out absolutely.

Nutrition:

Keto Bagels Recipe (low carb)

Amount per Serving

245 Calories, Calories from Fat 189

Value on a daily basis

Carbohydrates 6g 2%

Protein 12g 24%

Fat 21g is 32%

Fiber 3g 13%

Sodium 316mg 14%

Nutrition facts:

Sodium: 316mg | Calories: 245kcal | Protein: 12g | Fat: 21g | Carbohydrates: 6g | Fiber: 3g

3.3 Keto Sausage and Egg Breakfast Sandwich

Cook your eggs in the circle of a Mason jar lid to make those perfectly round-shaped eggs. You can also get egg molds with silicone to do the trick.

Prep Time: 5 minutes, Yield: Makes 1 serving, Cook Time: 10 minutes, Total Time: 15 minutes

Ingredients:

- 1 tbsp butter
- 1 tbsp mayonnaise
- 2 slices sharp cheddar cheese
- 2 large eggs
- A few slices of avocado
- 2 sausage patties, cooked

Instructions:

Heat the butter over medium pressure, in a large skillet. Place lightly oiled molds of silicone eggs or rings of Mason jar into the pan.

Then crack the eggs in the loops, then use a fork to crack the yolks, then whisk softly — cover and cook for over 3-4 minutes, or until eggs have been cooked. Remove the ringed eggs.

Place one of the eggs on your plate and top half the mayonnaise over it. Place one of the sausage patties on top of the egg.

Cover the patty sausage with a cheese slice and an avocado.

Put the second patty sausage over the avocado and then top it with your remaining cheese.

Spread the leftover mayonnaise over the second cooked egg and place over the cheese.

Serve, and have fun.

Recipe Notes:

6g net carbs per Serving

If you want to decrease the fat content and calories, you can skip the butter and omit the mayonnaise.

Nutrition:

Fiber: 2g, Calories: 880, Fat: 82g, Serving Size: 1 Breakfast Sandwich, Carbohydrates: 8g, Protein: 32g

3.4 Bacon &Egg Breakfast Wraps with Avocado

Cheddar cheese, bacon & eggs, salsa, and avocado fill those breakfast wraps. This low carb, as well as the extremely easy recipe, keeps you full every morning.

Servings: 2, Course: Breakfast, Prep Time: 5 minutes, Cook Time: 10 minutes, Cuisine: American, Total Time: 15 minutes, Calories: 469kcal

Ingredients:

- 1/4 cup salsa
- 2 Almost Zero Carb Wraps
- 2 large eggs
- 1/2 cup grated cheddar cheese

- 3 slices of bacon cooked
- 1/2 avocado sliced
- Salt and pepper to taste

Instructions:

Cook your bacon in the frying pan until it is crisp. Remove, halve, and set aside. Measure out all but 2 pork fat Teaspoons. Cut the avocado.

Beat the eggs in a tiny bowl and half the cheddar cheese with a pick. To your preference, cook the scrambled eggs and extract them from the pot—season with pepper and salt.

Place the wraps over medium heat within the hot pan. Portion the scrambled eggs and then place them on half of each wrap, not passing midway through. Attach the ham, avocado, and the leftover cheese. Add 1 spoonful of water to the pot and immediately cover with a seal. Leave it covered with a lid for 1-2 minutes or covered until your cheese has melted and a little browned at the lower part of the wraps. Serve on salsa.

Nutrition Facts:

Bacon & Egg Breakfast Wraps with Avocado (Keto)

Amount per Serving

Calories 469Calories from Fat 342

% Daily Value*

Carbohydrates 4g 1%

Fat 38g 58%

Protein 27g 54%

Fiber 1g 4%

Nutrition:

Fat: 38g | Calories: 469kcal | Protein: 27g | Carbohydrates: 4g | Fiber: 1g

3.5 Low Carb Stuffed Zucchini Boats (Gluten-Free)

These Zucchini Breakfast Vessels, loaded with scrambled eggs and sausage, are a perfect gluten-free and low carb way to have a serving of veggies at your morning meal.

Servings: 4, Cuisine: American, Prep Time: 10 minutes, Course: Breakfast, Cook Time: 20 minutes, Total Time: 30 minutes, Calories: 537kcal

Ingredients:

- Zucchini Boat Shells
- Salt and pepper to taste
- Sausage Filling
- 2 ounces onion chopped
- 16 ounces zucchini or Magda squash 2-3 squashes
- 1-ounce green bell pepper chopped
- 1 clove garlic minced
- 1/4 teaspoon dried thyme
- 1/8 teaspoon dried sage
- 8 ounces sausage
- Scrambled Eggs
- 4 large eggs
- 3 ounces cheddar cheese
- 2 tablespoons butter
- 1/2 cup salsa

Instructions:

Preparation: Cut the courgette in half and scrape the center, leaving a good, firm "cover." Put a stable glass baking dish in a microwave and cover it with plastic wrap. Cook for 4-5 minutes at high strength, just until cooked through. In the meantime, chop the onions, green bell, garlic, and pepper. Roll the cheese.

Cook: Add the onion, garlic, and pepper in a large saute pan and then cook until it begins to turn translucent, and then push the veggies to the side and place the sausage in the center of the pan, flatten it out so that it can brown. Sprinkle over the sausage with sage and thyme. Flip the sausage when browned, and start breaking it, mixing it with the bell pepper and onions. Totally cook the sausage. Take off the pan and cover to stay dry. Assemble: Flame a non-stick pan over medium heat and heat the butter before foaming ends. In the meanwhile, bring the eggs into a blender and combine on small. Put the eggs into the pan when the butter is soft, and scramble. Switch off the oven and add the vegetables and sausage and pour in the scrambled eggs. Sprinkle 3/4th of the cheese on the sausage and top with scrambled eggs before the cheese melts. Season the zucchini boats with pepper and salt, then divide the filling between them and then top up the cheese.

Put the cheese in the oven, or under your broiler to melt— season with salsa.

Nutrition Facts:

Low Carb Stuffed Zucchini Boats for Breakfast (Gluten-Free)

Amount per Serving (1 g)

Calories 537Calories from Fat 423

% Daily Value

Fiber 2g 8%

Fat 47g7 2%

Protein 22g 44%

Carbohydrates 8g 3%

Nutrition:

Serving: 1g | Carbohydrates: 8g | Protein: 22g | Calories: 537kcal | Fat: 47g | Fiber: 2g

3.6 Caesar Salad Deviled Eggs

Yield: 4 Servings (3 Deviled Eggs)

Ingredients:

- 1/3 cup creamy caesar dressing
- Cracked black pepper, to taste
- 1/2 cup Parmesan cheese, shredded, divided
- 6 large pastured eggs, hard-boiled, peeled and halved
- 1 romaine lettuce leaf, shredded

Instructions:

Fork mix the egg yolks into a mixing pot. Add 1/4th cup Parmesan cheese, Caesar dressing, and half lettuce shredded. Mix well before mixed.

Using a pastry bag to pipe the mix back into the eggs.

Put a little Parmesan cheese, black pepper, and shredded lettuce on top of each egg.

Nutrition:

Serving Size: Protein: 13.5g, 254, Carbohydrates: 2.75g, Fat: 22g

3.7 Bacon-Wrapped Scotch Eggs with Hollandaise and Asparagus

Ingredients:

- 6 large eggs
- 4 slices thick-cut bacon
- 1-pound bulk Italian sausage
- 1 cup sharp cheddar cheese, shredded
- 1 bundle asparagus
- 1 batch keto hollandaise

Directions:

Put eggs in the water and fill a moderate saucepan with some cold water. Bring water over high heat to a rolling boil. Remove the heat from the pan, cover, and leave it as it is for 10 minutes. Run the eggs and peel under cold water. Preheat your oven to 400 ° C, add cheese and sausage in a wide mixing dish. Divide the mixture into 6 portions, which are equal. The sections are cut out into patties. Then place an egg over every sausage patty and then form the sausage again around the egg until fully covered. Place a refrigerating rack on the top of the baking sheet and then line your bacon strips on it. Place the eggs wrapped in sausage on the rack, too. Bake for 30 minutes. Before eating, wrap every Scotch egg with a bacon strip.

Prep Time: 20 Minutes

Makes Servings: 6

Cook Time: 30 Minutes

Nutrition:

Per Serving:

Protein – 26 g

Carbs – 2 net g

Calories – 423

Fat – 35 g

3.8 Creamy Herbed Bacon and Egg Skillet

This rich in cream and herbs Bacon and Egg Skillet certainly spice up the routine for breakfasts. A one-pot meal that is so delicious and simple to put together.

Prep Time: 10 minutes, Yield: 4 servings, Cook Time: 15 minutes, Total Time: 25 minutes

Ingredients:

- 1/4 cup feta cheese, crumbled
- 1 tsp garlic powder
- 1/2 cup heavy cream
- 2 tbsp Italian flat-leaf parsley
- 2 tbsp fresh chives, chopped
- 1/4 cup sour cream
- 1 tbsp fresh dill
- 1 tsp onion powder
- Cracked black pepper, to taste
- 8 large eggs
- 1 tsp sea salt, more to taste
- 6 slices bacon, cooked crisp and crumbled

Instructions:

Preheat your oven to 425 ° C

Merge heavy cream, parsley, garlic powder, chives, dill, onion powder, sour cream, pepper, and marine salt in a big, ovenproof frying pan. At medium-low heat, put to a steady boil.

The eggs crack into the frying pan. Place the skillet into the oven. Then bake your eggs until the egg-whites have been set well, and the yolks of eggs have reached the level of completeness desired.

Remove from oven and then sprinkle over the top with chopped feta and bacon.

Nutrition:

Serving Size: 1/4 of the skillet, Protein: 18g, Fat: 31g, Carbohydrates: 3.75g, Calories: 362

3.9 Pizza Eggs (Low Carb, Keto, Gluten-Free)

When you have had Pizza Eggs, you will get hooked automatically. These put pizza as a totally appropriate breakfast choice on the table. This takes comparatively longer than cooking the eggs usually; however, the end product would be worthwhile.

Yield: Makes1 Serving

Ingredients:

- 5 slices pepperoni
- 1 tablespoon butter or olive oil
- 2 tablespoons Pizza Sauce
- 1 tablespoon grated parmesan cheese
- 2 large eggs
- 2 tablespoons mozzarella cheese, shredded
- Dash Italian seasoning

Instructions:

Heat butter over medium-low heat in an egg-pan. (You don't need to use an egg pan particularly, but if you use it makes it easier.)

Crack the eggs into your pan until the butter is warmed, and the water is warm.

When the whites have just begun settling and becoming green, drizzle some sauce onto the eggs then scatter the feta over it.

Reduce heat to small, and cook away. Put mozzarella cheese, Italian seasoning, pepperoni, and on top until the whites are nearly fully finished.

Start cooking on low heat until the whites are fully set, the cheese gets melted, and the pepperoni gets cooked

Nutrition:

Carbohydrates: 5.5g, Calories: 397, Sodium: 547mg, Fat: 31.8g, Sugar: 1.4g, Saturated Fat: 16.1g, Protein: 20.8g

3.10 Eggs Keto Benedict Casserole

Cook Time: 20 minutes, Preparation Time: 10 Minutes, Total Time: 30 mins, Yield: 6 Servings

Ingredients:

- 1/4 tsp black pepper
- 12 ounces thinly sliced ham
- 1/4 teaspoon paprika
- 10 large pastured eggs
- 1 tablespoon butter or olive oil
- 2 tablespoons Dijon mustard
- 1 teaspoon onion powder

- 1/2 cup heavy cream
- 1 teaspoon garlic powder
- 1/4 teaspoon sea salt
- 1 Batch of Keto Hollandaise Sauce

Instructions:

Preheat your oven to 350 degrees F.

Set 6 Canadian bacon slices aside, and then chop the others which are rest.

Heat up the butter over medium flame high heat in a big skillet. When the butter has melted, add up the Canadian bacon, and your pan is hot. Cook until just beginning to brown.

Then crack your eggs and whisk into a mixing bowl of large size. Stir in heavy cream, onion powder, sea salt, mustard Dijon, garlic powder, paprika, and black pepper. Then whisk until all the ingredients have mixed well. Add in 3/4 of the fried Canadian bacon.

A line on the lower end of an 8x13 baking dish the remaining six loaves of Canadian bacon.

Spurt the egg mixture on the Canadian bacon sliced on top.

Bake for another 20 minutes. And then, remove the leftover Canadian bacon from the oven and then sprinkle over the top.

Back towards the oven, then bake for another 10 minutes.

Until eating, top up with sauce named hollandaise.

Nutrition:

2g net carbs by per Serving

Calories: 280, Carbohydrates: 2g, Fat: 21g, Protein: 20g

3.11 Corned Beef Hash Breakfast Skillet (Paleo, Low Carb)

This Skillet Corned Beef Hash Breakfast is the best way to continue the day. A healthy meal of cauliflower hash, pastured eggs, and corned beef, both cooked to perfection.

Yield: 4 Servings, Cooking Time needed: 25 minutes, Total Time: 30 minutes, Prep Time: 5 minutes.

Ingredients:

- 4 large pastured eggs
- 2 tbsp olive oil
- 3 cloves garlic, minced
- 2 cups riced cauliflower
- 1 medium onion, diced
- 1 lb. corned beef, diced
- 2 tbsp Italian flat-leaf parsley, rough chopped
- 1/4 cup Russian dressing

Instructions:

Over medium flame, warm the olive oil in a pan.

Add garlic and onion to the frying pan. Sauté until translucent onion, and garlic gives fragrant.

Attach the cauliflower, which is riced and sauté until partially caramelized and cooked clean.

The corned beef is applied to the skillet. Saute, frequently stirring until the corned beef crisps up.

Make four wells in the corned beef combination, using a large spoon. Make them quite deep enough to expose the bottom of the pan. Crack each well into an egg. Reduce heat to medium-low, and allow cooking through the eggs.

Sprinkle Russian dressing with fresh parsley and then drizzle on the top of the frying pan before serving.

Nutrition:

5.5g net carbs per Serving

Protein: 23g, Calories: 407, Carbohydrates: 7g, Fat: 32g, Fiber: 1.5g

3.12 Italian Spaghetti Casserole Squash

Yield: Makes 4 Servings

Ingredients:

- 2 cloves garlic, minced
- 1 big spaghetti squash, seeded and lengthwise
- Sea salt and black pepper, to taste
- 1/2 tsp dried Italian seasoning
- 1 cup onion, diced
- 4 tbsp butter, ghee or bacon fat, divided
- 3 oz Italian salami, sliced
- 4 large eggs
- 1/2 cup organic tomatoes, diced
- A handful of Italian flat-leaf parsley, chopped
- 1/2 cup kalamata olives, halved

Directions:

Heat your oven 400 ° Put halves of spaghetti squash on a baking sheet which is rimmed, cut side up. Place 1 tbsp of butter on every half of it. Generously sprinkle with black pepper and salt. Bake for a single hour or until tender for 45 minutes.

While when you are baking the squash spaghetti, warm up a frying pan over medium flame low heat, which is ovenproof. Add the leftover 2 tbsp butter to the saucepan. Add the sea salt, onions, garlic, and pepper to the saucepan once your butter is melted.

Once your onions have begun caramelizing, add the salami and tomatoes. Saute for another 10 minutes, then mix up in the olives of the kalamata.

Once roasting is done with the squash spaghetti, use a fork for scraping the flesh out of both halves. Then mix in the salami and onion mixture with the spaghetti squash.

Use a large-sized spoon in the blend to create four deep wells. Crack each well into an egg.

Place the saucepan into your oven and then bake until the egg whites are ready.

Before serving sprinkle with fresh parsley on the top.

Nutrition:

Fiber: 3.75 NET, Per Serving Calories: 333, Protein: 14g, Fat: 23g, Carbs: 17g, Net CARBS: 13.25g.

Chapter 4: Salty Light Bites for Keto Breakfast

This chapter will help you to learn and experiment with the different basic varieties of recipes that are used regularly in the snack timings or as your siders regarding the Ketogenic diet. These Keto snack recipes are exclusively for those who are on this diet, particularly or going for healthy and clean food.

4.1 Keto Bloomin' Onion:

Ingredients:

- 1/2 tbsp seasoning salt
- 1 cup pork rind breadcrumbs
- 1/2 tsp cayenne
- 1/2 tbsp paprika
- 1/2 cup coconut flour
- 1/2 tsp fresh ground pepper
- 4 tbsp heavy whipping cream
- 4 eggs
- 1 large sweet onion

Dipping Sauce:

- 5-10 dashes of hot sauce
- 3/4 cup full-fat sour cream
- 1 tsp paprika
- 1/2 tsp onion salt (or onion powder and salt can be used in its place)

Salt according to your taste, if need be.

Whisk all ingredients of the dipping sauce, until they are completely combined.

If possible, make it ahead of time, allowing flavors to mix. Store in the refrigerator to ready for use.

Directions:

Cut the onion 1/4 off the top and, at the bottom, leave the nub. Turn side down and then cut the onion in quarters, then 1/8, then sixteenth, leaving approximately 1/4 out of the nub.

Flip the onion over, and the middle petals (about the diameter of 1 inch) are sliced off.

Put coconut flour on the entire onion, removing petals and ensuring that everything, including the edges, is powdered.

Mix in a small bowl, the egg wash (heavy cream and eggs). Spoon 1/2 of egg, wash over the whole onion and make sure it gets in between petal and below until it is well covered. Don't be afraid to really use hands to get in there. It is important to stick the breadcrumbs on this.

Beat seasonings and breadcrumbs together in yet another tub. Place the onion into it and thoroughly coat it, making sure you get the bottom too. Turn over, and tap extra breadcrumbs.

Now repeat ... pour over breaded onion the second 1/2 of the egg wash and breadcrumbs. The back, front top and side of each petal should be coated.

Set onion carefully on the plate and place it in the refrigerator for one hour.

Add oil to a big heavy bottom pot (approx. two thirds full) and then heat to three hundred degrees. Lower onion carefully in hot oil with the nub side up for 1 minute

Lower to medium-low heat, and flip onion carefully, side up the petal. Carefully watching, let it fry for another two to three minutes.

Using large tongs to cut off the onion and let drain on a lined sheet of paper towel.

Serve alongside dipping sauce right away.

Nutrition Facts

Amount per Serving

Calories 71Calories from Fat 27

% Daily Value*

Fat 3g5%

Saturated Fat 1g6%

Cholesterol 40mg13%

Sodium 105mg5%

Potassium 51mg1%

Carbohydrates 6g2%

Fiber 3g13%

Sugar 1g1%

Protein 2g4%

Vitamin A 360IU7%

Vitamin C 1mg1%

Calcium 9mg1%

Iron 0.5mg**3%**

Recipe Notes:

Pork rind "breadcrumbs" are far finer than the regular breadcrumbs, and you can hack onion petals off with a tiny knife instead of cutting off as you might in the initial recipe.

Air fryer should not be used to cook this.

4.2 Lettuce Wraps (With Keto Hoisin Sauce)

Total time: 40 minutes

Yield: 8 servings

Cook time: 15 minutes

Prep time: 25 minutes

Ground turkey is sprinkled with a savory and sweet low-carbohydrates sesame ginger sauce and presented inside butter cups for delightful Asian-inspired food.

Ingredients:

For the Sauce:

- 1 tablespoon almond butter, natural
- 2 cloves garlic, minced
- 3 tablespoons less-sodium soy sauce
- 1/2 teaspoon ginger paste
- 1 tablespoon rice vinegar
- 1 tablespoon sesame oil
- 1 tablespoon Swerve sweetener, brown
- For the Lettuce Wraps:
- 1/2 cup diced jicama
- 1-pound ground turkey
- 1 tablespoon olive oil
- 2 teaspoons dried minced onion
- 1/4 teaspoon salt
- 1/4 teaspoon pepper
- 3 oz. chopped shiitake mushrooms
- 3 green onions, thinly sliced
- Living butterhead lettuce

Directions:

In a small tub, whisk all the ingredients of the sauce, and put it aside.

Heat the olive oil to a frying pan on the stove. Crumble over medium heat, and cook the ground turkey—season with chopped onion, pepper a salt.

Add mushrooms, jicama, and green onion. Saute for 2 to 3 minutes with meat until the mushrooms become soft. Pour over meat sauce and combine.

Spoon the mixture on top of pieces of lettuce to serve. Enjoy it!

Recipe notes:

The recipe was made to fill about four cups. 1/4 cup for one wrap that will make 16 wraps of lettuce in total.

Nutritional Information:

Yield: Serving Size: 2 wraps, 16 lettuce wraps, (1/4 cup for one wrap)

Fiber: 2g, Net Carbohydrates: 2.5g, Sugar Alcohols: 1.5g, Total Fat: 9g. Amount per Serving: Protein: 12g, Total Carbohydrates: 6g, Calories: 149.

4.3 Keto Chili

Prep time: 15 minutes

Yield: 8 servings

Total time: 1 hour 45 minutes

Cook time: 1 hour 30 minutes

A low form of carbohydrate that truly curbs cravings.

Ingredients:

- 1/2 teaspoon black pepper
- 2/3 cups celery, finely diced
- 3 pounds ground beef (I use 85/15), drained, reserving 2 tbsp of fat
- 1/2 cup red bell pepper
- 1 1/2 cups yellow onion
- 1/2 cup green bell pepper
- 1 1/2 cups tomato juice
- 1 cup tomatoes, finely chopped

- 1 1/2 teaspoons Worcestershire sauce
- 15 oz can crushed tomatoes in puree
- 2 teaspoons erythritol, granular
- 3 tablespoons chili powder
- 1 teaspoon garlic powder
- 1 teaspoon salt
- 1/2 teaspoon oregano
- 1 teaspoon cumin

Directions:

Brown your ground beef in a big pot just until done. Drain much of the fat and leave only two spoonsful.

Add the celery, onions, bell pepper, and tomatoes to the beef pot. Keep cooking for another 5 minutes over medium to high heat.

Now add the crushed tomatoes, tomato juice, Worcestershire sauce, and all of the seasonings. Cover the pot, stirring regularly, and boil for one to one and a half hours.

Recipe notes:

10 min before serving remove and uncover from heat. Cover with the minced cheddar cheese, and at last diced onions if needed. Enjoy it!

Nutritional information:

Amount per Serving: Total Carbohydrates: 11, Calories: 344, Fiber: 2, Total Fat: 21, Net Carbohydrates: 9Protein: 27

Yield: 8 servings

4.4 Low Carb Keto Biscuits

Prep time: 10 minutes, Servings: 9 biscuits, Cooking time: 10 minutes, Course: appetizer, Total time: 20 minutes, Cuisine: American

These soft drops and tender biscuits can be ready in 30 min. You're not going to skip a meal in any way. The biscuits really are keto-free gluten-free and are low carbohydrate.

Ingredients:

- 1/2 cup shredded cheddar cheese
- ¼ tsp. salt
- 1½ cups superfine almond flour
- 1 tbsp baking powder
- ½ tsp onion powder
- ½ tsp garlic powder
- 2 large eggs
- 4 tbsp unsalted butter melted
- 1/2 cup sour cream

Instructions:

Preheat the oven to 450 ° F. A 12-cup muffin pan grease the muffin fillings lightly.

Whisk the onion powder, almond flour, garlic powder, baking powder, and salt together in a big bowl.

Combine the eggs, sour cream, and butter in a small bowl. Whisk to smoothness. Pour the dry ingredients into a large bowl.

Mix with a spoon until the mixture of the batter is even. It will be pretty dense. Add cheese.

Add 1/4 cup of butter in the mold of muffin. The batter can be sticky, so you shall probably need to scrape with a spatula and remove the entire batter from the measuring cup. Repeat till all the batters are used

Bake the biscuits for about 10 to 11 min or until the top of biscuits are golden brown, and the inserted toothpick comes to clean out of them. Before eating slightly, cool the biscuits.

Recipe notes:

Baking this one in a muffin tin is better since your batter is really moist, so if you attempt to cook them free on a baking surface, it will spill out too far.

Using full-fat cream cheese is the secret to the soft and luxurious feel. You can also add cheese cream or simple Greek yogurt if you don't have some sour cream at your house, though.

Today's recipe is for savory biscuits with cheese. But by putting herbs (thyme, rosemary, chives, parsley are great choices) in the batter or by switching cheese for another cheese, change can easily be made.

Nutrition:

Serving: 1biscuit: carbohydrates: 5g, calories: 216kcal, protein: 7g, saturated fat: 6g, fat: 19g, cholesterol: 63mg, potassium: 172mg, sodium: 129mg, fiber: 2g, vitamin a: 355iu, sugar: 1g, calcium: 163mg, vitamin c: 0.1mg, net carbs: 3g iron: 1mg.

4.5 Low-Carb Zuppa Toscana Soup

Cook time: 20 minutes

Prep time: 20 minutes

Total time: 40 minutes

Yield: 6 servings

Ingredients:

- 1 cup heavy cream
- 1 onion, chopped
- 1-pound Italian sausage
- 3 cloves garlic, minced
- 1/4 teaspoon black pepper
- 1/2 teaspoon red pepper flakes
- 1/2 teaspoon salt

- 16 oz. chicken broth
- 1 head cauliflower, cut into florets
- 1-quart water
- 3 cups kale or Swiss chard, chopped
- 1 teaspoon bouillon

Directions:

Crumble and brown the sausage in a soup pot on the stove over medium to high heat.

Put the onion and garlic, and cook until color is translucent. Season it with salt flakes, vinegar, and red pepper.

Reduce the heat to medium. Add water, cauliflower florets, and broth. If necessary, mix in and apply bouillon.

Cook on a medium heat, about 15 to 20 minutes, until the cauliflower is soft.

Reduce to low heat and scatter with sliced kale. Pour the cream in, then stir well. Serve warm.

Nutritional information:

Amount per Serving: Total Carbohydrates: 15g, Calories: 450, Fiber: 3g, Total Fat: 37g, Net Carbohydrates: 12g, Protein: 18g

Serving Size: 1 serving, Yield: 6 servings

4.6 Keto Pickle-Brined Fried Chicken Bites with Sweet Mustard Sauce

Cook time: 20 minutes

Preparation time: 1 hour 20 minutes

Total time: 1 hour 40 minutes

Yield: 4 servings

This recipe of keto fried chicken won't leave you on the spot in only a few quick steps.

Ingredients:

For mustard sauce:

- 10-15 drops liquid stevia (according to your taste as many stevia brands vary in sweetness)
- 2 teaspoons of dijon mustard
- 1/2 cup mayonnaise
- 2 teaspoons of apple cider vinegar
- 1/4 teaspoon turmeric
- 1/2 teaspoon of garlic powder
- 1/4 teaspoon of onion powder

For Chicken:

- 1 to 2 cups pickle juice
- 1-pound chicken breast, sliced into 1-inch pieces
- 1/2 teaspoon salt
- 1 tablespoon baking powder
- 1/2 cup of unflavored whey protein isolate
- 1 tablespoon of confectioners, erythritol
- 1/2 teaspoon of garlic powder
- 1/2 to 1 teaspoon salt
- 1/2 teaspoon paprika
- Oil, high flame tolerant
- 1/2 teaspoon black pepper

Directions:

The mustard:

Mix dijon mustard, mayonnaise, garlic powder sugar, turmeric, stevia, and onion powder together in a medium cup, until well mixed. Place in or cover with a container and set aside till bites of chicken are ready to eat.

(Mustard sauce may be refrigerated in a sealed bag for up to 2 weeks.)

The chicken

In a shallow dish or Ziplock bag, place the cubed shaped chicken, then add the kosher salt and the pickle juice. Mix well and ensure all pieces of chicken are soaked in the pickle brine. Put the chicken in a fridge for 30-60 minutes to marinate. Remove the chicken to room temperature from the fridge for about 25 mins before frying. This contributes to promoting even superior texture and cooking.

Pat the chicken pieces drain and dry your brine and until they are marinated. Set aside.

To fry pan:

Place a wide frying pan with a high side over moderate to moderate/low flame. Pour oil into a saucepan to establish a sufficient 1/2-inch oil volume. Using a thermometer and maintain the temperature of the oil at about 350 degrees for better performance. (If the oil becomes very hot, the butter may melt. Instead, if the oil is not very hot, the batter may consume extra oil and will not crisp up well.)

To deep-fry:

Turn on the fryer and set temperature to approximately 350 degrees (if you have a temperature gauge).

While oil gets heated, in a medium-low rimmed bowl, combine the whey protein powder, erythritol, baking powder, salt, paprika, garlic powder, and pepper. Blend well.

Place every chicken piece in the mixture till well coated on all sides. Put coated bites lined with the parchment paper on a saucepan or dish. Once all the pieces are covered, you may re-roll every other piece that requires extra coating till all of the mixtures are used up.

Drop bites of chicken into the hot oil and let it to fry for 4 to 6 mins or until it is cooked—flip half-way through cooking when pan-frying. The length depends on the temperature of the oil and the size of the chicken bite. Cut the cooking time into large chunks to test for doneness and gage. Put fried nuggets on a rack filled with paper towels to cool off.

Chicken is better consumed when hot and juicy right away. Serve with the light mustard sauce or the dipping sauces you want. Love it!

Recipe notes:

Heat the leftovers for about five minutes in a 350-degree hot oven or 3-5 minutes in the air fryer on 375-degree. This is not suggested that you microwave leftovers.

The main calorie information is only for chicken fried. Please note that the measurement of nutritional details contained a one-fourth cup of the avocado oil (to compensate for absorption).

Mustard sauce values are the following:

Serving size: approximately 1 tablespoon, Yield: 8 servings.

Amount per Serving: Carbohydrates: 0gram, Calories: 92, Fiber: 0gram, Fat: 10grams, Net Carbohydrates: 0gram, Protein: 0gram

Nutritional information:

Serving Size: 4 oz. of chicken bites, Yield: 4 servings

Amount per Serving: Total Carbohydrates: 3g, Calories: 284, Fiber: 0g, Net Carbohydrates: 1g, Sugar Alcohols: 2g, Protein: 34g, Total Fat: 17g

4.7 Turkey & Provolone

Prep time: 10 minutes

Yield: 1 serving

Total time: 10 minutes

This is how to create a healthy keto meal like the "Beach Party" turkey.

Ingredients:

For each unwich:

- 2-3 large pieces of iceberg lettuce
- 1 slice of provolone cheese, 1.5 oz.
- 2 pieces of sliced turkey, 2 oz.
- 3 slices of tomato, 1.5oz.
- 1/2 small avocado, 2 oz.
- 10 slices cucumber, 1.5 oz.
- Pinch salt
- 1 teaspoon real mayonnaise
- Pinch pepper
- 1 teaspoon yellow mustard

Directions:

Place 2-3 lettuce leaves in alternating lines.

Start with cheese and meat and lay all ingredients of the sandwich in the middle, however a bit closer to the bottom half of the lettuce. That will make the roll-up at the end easier. Wrap the lettuce tightly just as a burrito, i.e., folding each end in and then wrap tightly in a few squares of the parchment paper. Cover it using tape to cover, or a label.

Nutritional information:

Serving Size: 1 unwich, Yield: 1 serving.

Amount per Serving: Total Carbohydrates: 10, Calories: 359, Fiber: 6g, Total Fat: 26g, Net Carbohydrates: 4g, Protein: 22g

4.8 Keto Pepperoni Pizza Hot Pockets

Prep Time: 20 minutes, Total amount of Time: 40 minutes, Cooking Time: 20 minutes, Yield: 8 pizza pockets.

Ingredients:

FOR DOUGH:

- 1/2 teaspoon ground black pepper
- 5 tablespoons cream cheese
- 3 cups shredded low moisture, part-skim mozzarella cheese
- 2 large eggs
- 1 teaspoon garlic powder
- 2 cups blanched almond flour
- 1 teaspoon onion powder
- 1 teaspoon of sea salt
- 1 teaspoon Italian seasoning

FOR FILLING:

- 2 cups shredded sharp white cheddar cheese
- 1 large egg, whisked
- 5 ounces sliced pepperoni (about 48 slices)
- 1/2 cup Paleo Pizza Sauce

Instructions:

Preheat oven to 425 ° F

Mix the cream cheese and the mozzarella in a broad microwave protected mixing dish. Microwave it for 1 Minute. Remove it from the microwave, then mix to blend. Switch to the microwave for another 1 minute.

Add almond flour, eggs, garlic powder, onion powder, black pepper, Italian seasoning, and sea salt to mixing bowl. Blend before fully combined products are all liquid.

Divide your dough up into eight balls. Roll every ball up to 1/4-inch thickness between the two parchment paper sheets.

On each round, spoon one tablespoon of the pizza sauce and arrange it in a circle and leaving some space across the edges.

Place six pieces of your pepperoni and one-fourth cup of the cheddar cheese in the middle of each.

Brush the corners of dough with egg wash, then fold over and press to seal. Repeat with all eight pizza pockets this method.

Place pizza pockets on the baking sheet, and wash the brush egg over each of them.

Bake it for 20 minutes.

Nutrition:

Serving Size: 1 pizza pocket, Fat: 45.2g, Calories: 581, Carbohydrates: 11g, Protein: 36.2g, Fiber: 3g.

4.9 Keto Pizza Chips

Yield: 12 chips

Cooking Time: 15 minutes, Prep Time: 15 minutes, Total Time: 30 minutes,

Ingredients:

- Low Carbohydrates Pizza Sauce, optional for serving
- 1 teaspoon dried oregano
- 1 cup grated parmesan cheese
- 12 slices pepperoni

Instructions:

Preheat to 400 ° F on a burner. Line a parchment paper baking sheet, or even a silicone baking tray.

Spread your parmesan cheese over the baking tray in 12, even circles. They will be about one tablespoon, plus one teaspoon for each. Bake for another 2 minutes.

Remove the plate from your oven and sprinkle over the cheese with the oregano. Using one slice of pepperoni to cover every cheese circle and bake for an extra eight minutes, until its crisp.

Remove that tray from your oven, and dab each chip with a paper towel to soak excess grease.

Switch the chips to a cooling rack lined with a paper towel and encourage them to cool and keep crisping up.

Where desired, serve with the pizza sauce.

Nutrition:

Serving Size: 4 chips

Fat: 7.8g, Calories: 104 Carbohydrates: 0.7g Protein: 7.4g, Fiber: 0.1g

4.10 Buffalo Chicken Jalapeno Poppers

With this recipe, two popular bar appetizers recently got a big makeover. Instead of picking between buffalo chicken wings or jalapeno poppers, how about you, getting them in one platter? Talk about heaven made a match. Add some creamy dressing on the side of the ranch or blue cheese, and you're good to go.

Prep Time: 15 Minutes, Total Time required: 50 minutes, Cooking Time: 35 minutes, Yield: 5 (4 Poppers per serving), Cuisine: Keto, Low Carb, Appetizer, Gluten-free.

Ingredients:

- 2 green onions, sliced, for garnish
- 8 ounces ground chicken

- 10 large jalapeño peppers, halved lengthwise and seeded
- 2 cloves garlic, minced
- ½ teaspoon fine sea salt
- ½ teaspoon onion powder
- ½ cup crumbled blue cheese, divided
- 4 ounces cream cheese (½ cup), softened
- ¼ cup shredded mozzarella cheese
- 4 strips bacon, cooked crisp and crumbled
- ¼ cup buffalo wing sauce
- For serving, ranch dressing

Instructions:

Preheat to 350 ° F on the oven. Cover the ringed baking sheet with the baking mat or parchment paper or silicone. Spread the halves of jalapeño over the baking sheet.

Over medium heat, large heat skillet. Attach the meat, ginger, onion powder, and sea salt to the pan.

Saute until chicken is not pink anymore and then cook all the way. Move the fried chicken to a large mixing bowl. Add your cream cheese, Buffalo wing sauce mozzarella cheese, and 1/4 cup of the crumbled blue sticks.

Mix when all the components are blended properly.

Fill every jalapeno with a mixture of chicken mounds – top with remaining 1/4 cup of crumbling blue cheese, as well as bacon.

Bake for thirty minutes, until golden brown, is on top.

Before serving, top off with green onions.

Recipe notes:

If you can't seem to find the ground chicken in your local supermarket, just feel free to replace ground turkey.

Nutrition:

Serving Size: 4 poppers, Fat: 19g, Calories: 252, Carbohydrates: 4.6g, Protein: 16g, Fiber: 1g.

4.11 Cajun Trinity Keto Crab Cakes

The recipe yields eight very big, entrée-sized patties. You can easily get sixteen out of the recipe if you prepare smaller patties.

Yield: 8 Crab Cakes, Prep Time: 15 minutes, Total Time: 35 minutes, Cook Time: 20 minutes

Ingredients:

- 1 teaspoon spicy brown mustard
- 1 rib celery, finely chopped
- 2 tablespoons butter
- 1/2 cup mixed bell pepper, chopped
- 2 cloves of garlic, minced
- 1 teaspoon hot sauce
- 1 shallot, chopped
- Black pepper and sea salt, to taste
- 2 tablespoons of mayonnaise
- 1 large egg
- 1/2 cup crushed pork rinds
- 1/2 cup Parmesan cheese, grated
- 2 tablespoons olive oil
- 1-pound lumped crabmeat
- 1 tablespoon Worcestershire sauce

Instructions:

Heat up a large, sauté pan on medium flame. In the oven, heat the butter and add the sea salt, shallot, bell pepper, black pepper garlic. Stir, for about ten minutes, until your vegetables are moist and translucent.

In a big mixing bowl, add the squash, mayonnaise, light brown mustard, Worcestershire, and hot sauce. Stir in your sautéed vegetables. Mix until well added. Mix with the rinds of pork and Parmesan cheese. Fold the blend over your crab.

With a rimmed baking sheet or parchment, line a large plate. Form the mixture of your crabs into 8 similarly shaped patties — place patties on the baking sheet that you have prepared and refrigerated for 1-2 hrs.

Put some olive oil in a fry pan, in a big skillet on a medium-high flame, until your crab cakes are crispy and golden brown on either side. Be watchful that you do not turn them over so many times, or break them apart.

Nutrition:

Serving Size: 2 Crab Cakes, Fat: 28g, Calories: 412, Carbohydrates: 4g, Protein: 35g, Fiber: 1g

4.12 Crispy Baked Garlic Parmesan Wings

Yield: 6 servings, Cooking Time needed: 1 hour 15 minutes, Prep Time: 10 minutes, plus 20 minutes rest time, Total Time: 1 hour 45 minutes,

Ingredients:

- 1/4 teaspoon ground black pepper
- 1 teaspoon of sea salt
- 2 pounds chicken wings, thawed if frozen
- 2 tablespoons baking powder
- 1/2 cup grated Parmesan cheese
- 1/2 cup salted butter, melted
- 1 clove garlic, minced
- 1 1/2 teaspoons garlic powder
- 1 tablespoon chopped fresh flat-leaf parsley
- 1/2 teaspoon onion powder

Instructions:

Spread the wings over few paper towels in a single pan, then sprinkle with oil. Cover with a different paper towel layers and allow to rest for twenty minutes.

Place the oven rack in the middle-lower position and some other rack in place mid-upper. Preheat to 250 ° F on the oven. Set a tray on the rimmed baking sheet for cooling.

Combine wings in the resalable plastic container with baking powder. Shake to coat evenly on the wings.

Spread the wings across the refrigerating rack in a single layer—Bake for 30 minutes on the medium-lower oven rack.

Increase the heat to 425 ° F, and transfer your baking sheet to the middle-upper shelf. Bake your wings for another 45 minutes or until the skin is crispy and nice.

Mix the Parmesan cheese, onion powder, melted butter, garlic powder, minced garlic, pepper, and parsley in a medium dish, when the wings are frying, render the sauce.

Remove your wings from your oven, and require 5 minutes of rest. Before serving, stir in the sauce.

Nutrition:

Serving Size: 1/6th, Fat: 38g, Calories: 468Carbohydrates: 2g, Protein: 30g, Fiber: 0g,

4.13 Keto Popcorn Chicken

Prep Time: 15 minutes, Cooking Time needed: 20 minutes, Total Time: 35 minutes, Yield: 4 servings

Ingredients:

- 1 cup buttermilk
- 1-pound boneless, skinless chicken breasts, cut into bite-sized pieces
- ¼ cup coconut flour
- 1/8 teaspoon ground black pepper

- ½ teaspoon smoked paprika
- 1/4 teaspoon sea salt
- 1 large egg
- 1 teaspoon onion powder
- 2 cups crushed pork rinds
- ½ teaspoon garlic powder

Instructions:

PREVIOUS DAY:

Place the cut-up chicken in a pot, pour over the buttermilk, cover and cool for 24 hours.

NEXT DAY:

Preheat to 425 ° F on the oven. Top a parchment paper rimmed baking dish or silicone baking pad.

Have 3 shallow bowls set up. The salt, coconut flour, and pepper are combined in the first bowl. Crack the egg in the second tub then whisk the fork. The garlic powder, pork rinds, paprika, and onion powder mix together in the 3rd bowl.

With every piece of chicken, follow the following three-step process: dredge in the coconut flour, then you coat in the egg wash, then coat in breading pork rind. Place every breaded piece over the prepared baking sheet in a single line.

Boil for about 20 minutes, regularly checks, or until crispy and golden brown.

Nutrition:

Fiber: 1.5g, Fat: 13g, Calories: 466, Carbohydrates: 6.1g, Protein: 63g

4.14 Low Carb Keto Pizza Bagels

Yield: 6 Pizza Bagels, Prep Time: 15 minutes, Total Time: 29 minutes, Cooking Time: 14 minutes,

Ingredients:

- 1 tablespoon baking powder
- 2 cups almond flour
- 1 teaspoon garlic powder
- 1 teaspoon dried Italian seasoning
- 1 teaspoon onion powder
- 2 large eggs, whisked
- 2 tablespoons shredded Parmesan cheese
- 3 tablespoons cream cheese
- 3 cups shredded low moisture mozzarella cheese
- 1/4 cup Low Carb Pizza Sauce
- 1 teaspoon dried oregano
- 2.5 ounces pepperoni slices, chopped

Instructions:

Preheat oven to 425 F. Line a parchment paper rimmed on a baking sheet or a Silpat.

Combine the almond flour, baking powder, onion powder, garlic powder, and dry Italian seasoning in a medium mixing bowl. Mix well until combined. Run the mixture through the flour sifter to ensure sure all the baking powder is combined with the rest of the ingredients.

Combine the cream cheese and the mozzarella cheese in a big microwave-safe mixing bowl. Microwave it for about 1 minute and 30 seconds. Remove from the microwave, and combine to stir. Return the bowl to microwave for 30 secs at a time if needed, until the cheese is completely melted and easily mixed. Mix well until combined.

Apply the eggs and almond flour blend to the mixing pot. Mix before fully combined products are all in. If the dough becomes unworkable and too stringy, simply put it all back in the microwave to soften and then continue mixing for 30 seconds.

When it is well balanced, apply the pepperoni to your dough and blend in. Add and mix in the sauce, slowly. The dough here should be very fluffy.

Divide the dough into 6 parts, which are similar. Wrap each piece into a disk.

Press your finger gently into the center of every ball of dough to form a ring. Stretch out the ring to form a small hole in the middle into the bagel shape.

Top every other bagel with Parmesan and Oregano

Bake for 12-15 minutes or until the color is golden brown.

Nutrition:

Serving Size: 1 bagel, Calories: 449, Fat: 35g, Carbohydrates: 10g, Fiber: 4g, Protein: 28g

4.15 Keto Cauliflower Poppers Pizza

Yield=6 servings, Cook Time=30 minutes, Prep Time=15 minutes, Total Time=45 minutes

Ingredients:

- 2 tablespoons butter or olive oil, melted
- 1 large cauliflower head, cut and trimmed into florets
- 1/4 teaspoon sea salt or add more to taste
- 3 large dried tomatoes that are finely chopped
- 1 (14.5 ounces) can diced tomatoes
- 1 clove garlic that is minced
- 1.5 ounces hard chorizo that is finely chopped
- 1 small red bell pepper, finely chopped
- 1 tablespoon fresh basil
- 1 cup white cheddar cheese, shredded sharp
- 1/4 teaspoon ground black pepper

Instructions:

Preheat to about 400 ° F on the oven. Line your rimmed parchment-papered baking sheet.

Arrange your cauliflower florets over the baking sheet in one single layer. Drizzle over the top of your melted butter, sprinkle with the salt, and toss it to coat.

On the top rack, roast your cauliflower for 15 minutes.

Heat a big saucepan on medium while cauliflower is being roasted. Add the onions, sun-dried onions, garlic, chorizo, basil, bell pepper, and black pepper to the plate. When the sauce gets hot and begins bubbling gently, reduce heat to medium or low and simmer for ten minutes. Switch the sauce to the high-powered blender or the food processor, then a quick pump. Alternatively, this stage may be skipped and left to curvy. Pour your sauce on cauliflower and continue to roast for another 10 minutes, then remove the plate from your oven, scatter over the cheese, and bake it for another ten minutes or until cheese has melted.

Nutrition:

Fat=13.7g, Calories=196, Fiber=4.5g, Carbohydrates=11.2g, Protein=9.6g

4.16 Buffalo Chicken Egg Muffins (Low Carb, Gluten-Free)

Yield: Makes 4 Servings, Preparation Time: 15 minutes, Total Time: 35 minutes, Cook Time: 20 minutes,

Ingredients:

- 6 oz chicken, cooked and chopped
- 8 large eggs
- ¼ cup blue cheese crumbles (omit the cheese to make it paleo)
- 2 green onions, chopped
- 3 tbsp Buffalo Wing Sauce

- 1 rib celery, chopped
- Sea salt and black pepper, to taste
- 1 clove garlic, minced

Instructions:

Preheat oven for about 350 °. Oil lightly your muffin tin.

Fork whisk the eggs into a mixing bowl. Add the chicken, crumbles of blue cheese, green onions, garlic, buffalo-wing sauce, sea salt celery, and pepper to the eggs. Mix ingredients until fully incorporated into each other.

Pour the blend into the muffin tin, and that would serve to fill 8 spaces.

Bake it for twenty minutes, or until the top is brunette as well as golden brown.

Nutrition:

Fat: 11g | Per Serving – Calories: 238 | Carbs: 2.5g |Protein: 27g

Serving Size: 2 Egg Muffins Fat: 11g, Calories: 238,

4.17 Keto Soft Pretzel

Yield: Makes 6 pretzels, Prep Time: 15 minutes, Total Time: 29 minutes, Cooking Time: 14 minutes,

Ingredients:

- 5 tablespoons cream cheese
- 1 tablespoon baking powder
- 2 cups blanched almond flour
- Coarse sea salt, for topping
- 1 teaspoon garlic powder
- 3 large eggs, divided
- 1 teaspoon onion powder
- 3 cups shredded low moisture mozzarella cheese

Instructions:

First, heat the oven to 425 ° C. Line a parchment paper rimmed baking sheet or a Silpat.

The baking powder, almond flour, onion powder, and garlic powder are combined in the medium mixing bowl. Mix well until combined. Put the mixture over the flour sifter to make sure all your baking powder is mixed with all of the other ingredients and then crack one egg into a bowl and whisk in a fork. The egg wash for your top of the pretzels will be this. The other two eggs are going to go in the dough.

Combine the cream cheese and the mozzarella cheese in a safe microwave mixing bowl. Microwave for about 1 minute, 30 seconds, and then remove from the microwave, then mix to blend. Put it back into the microwave for an extra 1 minute. Mix well until combined.

Apply the additional 2 eggs and almond-flour mixture to the mixing pot. Mix all of the ingredients thoroughly. If the dough becomes unworkable and too stingy, simply place it back in your microwave to make it soft and continue mixing for 30 seconds.

Divide dough into 6 portions, which are equal. Roll every portion into a thin, long piece that resembles a breadstick. Fold every one of them into a pretzel shape.

Brush with the egg wash over the top of every pretzel.

Sprinkle on top of coarse sea salt.

Bake it for 12-14 minutes on the middle rack, or until they are golden brown.

Nutrition:

6g net carbohydrates per serving

Serving Size: 1 pretzel

Fat: 35.5g, Calories: 449, Fiber: 4g, Carbohydrates: 10g, Protein: 27.8g

4.18 Low Carb Chicken Pot Pie

4 Pot Pies = yield

Ingredients:

FOR POT PIE FILLING:

- 1/2 cup diced onion (about 2.5 oz)
- Salt and pepper, to taste
- 3 tbsp butter
- 1/2 cup celery, sliced
- 3 cloves of garlic, minced
- 1/2 cup carrots, sliced (about 2.5 oz)
- 3/4 cup heavy cream
- 1/2 cup chicken stock
- 12 oz chicken, cubed small
- 2 tbsp Dijon mustard
- 1/2 cup frozen peas
- 3/4 cup white cheddar cheese, shredded

FOR DOUGH:

- 1/2 tsp black pepper
- 3 tbsp cream cheese
- 1 1/2 cups mozzarella cheese, shredded
- 3/4 cup almond flour
- 1 tsp garlic powder
- 1 large egg
- 1 tsp onion powder
- 1 tsp sea salt
- 1 tsp Italian seasoning

Instructions:

FOR FILLING OF POT PIE:

Apply heat to butter on medium heat, into a large saucepan. Add the celery, onion, garlic, carrots, and a little pepper and salt to the saucepan when the butter melts. Sauce it until your vegetables are tender.

Add sauté and chicken to the saucepan until well cooked.

Add chicken stock, heavy cream, and mustard Dijon to the saucepan. Bring it to boil on medium-high heat, then reduce to low heat and allow it to simmer for 5 to 7 minutes.

Mix until melted, in the cheese.

Stir the peas in.

FOR DOUGH:

Preheat the oven until 375 ° C

Add cream cheese and mozzarella cheese in a large blending bowl. 1 Minute Microwave. Stir it to combine and add 1 additional minute to microwave. Mix in egg almond flour, Italian seasoning, garlic powder, onion powder, black pepper, and sea salt. Mix until all the ingredients have mixed well. If it gets stringy or it is not sufficiently melted, put it back in for more than 30 seconds.

Divide dough into 4 pieces, which are equal. Spread the pieces of dough out on Silpat or a parchment paper in large flat circles. If it starts getting sticky, then wet your hands a bit too so that it does not stick on you.

Divide the filling of the pot pie into large oven-safe ramekins or four mini-pin pans.

Top each with a piece of the dough and fold it over the edges.

Bake it for 20-25 minutes.

Nutrition:

Per Serving –Fat – 57g, Calories 661, Fiber – 4g, Protein – 43g, Net Carbs – 11g, Total Carbs – 15g

4.19 Low Carb Keto Everything Bagels

Yield: Makes 6 Bagels, Prep Time: 15 minutes, Total Time: 29 minutes, Cooking Time: 14 minutes,

Ingredients:

- 3 tablespoons Everything Bagel Seasoning
- 1 tablespoon baking powder
- 2 cups almond flour
- 1 teaspoon garlic powder
- 1 teaspoon dried Italian seasoning
- 1 teaspoon onion powder
- 3 large eggs, divided
- 5 tablespoons cream cheese
- 3 cups shredded low moisture mozzarella cheese

Instructions:

Preheat the oven to 425 ° C. Top a parchment paper rimmed baking dish, or a Silpat.

Combine the onion powder, baking powder, almond flour, garlic powder, and the Italian seasoning, which is dried in a small mixing dish. Mix well before mixed. Put the mixture into flour sifter to make sure all your baking powder is mixed with all the other ingredients, then crack one egg into a cup and mix with a pick. This will be the top-of-the-bagels egg wash. The remaining two eggs are going to go in the flour.

Combine the cream cheese and the mozzarella cheese in a large safe microwave mixing dish. Microwave for around 1.5 minutes, then remove from microwave, then mix to blend. Return to your microwave for another 1 minute. Mix well before mixed.

Apply the remaining two eggs and almond-flour mixture to the mixing pot. Mix all the ingredients until they are properly incorporated. If the dough is unworkable or too stingy, quickly bring it back to microwave to soften and start stirring for 30 seconds.

Divide your dough into 6 parts, which are equal. Wrap each piece in a ball shape.

Push your finger softly into the middle of a ball of dough to create a ring. Stretch out the ring to form a small hole into the center into a bagel form.

Brush each bagel's top with the wash of an egg.

Bake it for 12 to 14 minutes on the center rack, until its golden brown.

Nutrition:

6g net carbs per serving

Serving Size: 1 Bagel, Calories: 449, Fat: 35.5g, Carbohydrates: 10g, Fiber: 4g, Protein: 27.8g

4.20 Bacon Cheeseburger Pizza (Low Carb, Gluten-Free)

Yield= Makes 1 - 12 inches, pizza - 6 slices

Ingredients:

FOR CRUST:

- 3 tbsp cream cheese
- 1 1/2 cup mozzarella cheese, shredded
- 1 large egg
- 1/2 tsp black pepper
- 1 tsp garlic powder
- 3/4 cup almond flour
- 1 tsp Italian seasoning

- 1 tsp onion powder
- 1 tsp sea salt
- FOR TOPPINGS:
- 15 dill pickles slices
- 2 tsp yellow mustard
- 1/2 cup low carb pizza sauce
- 6 oz ground beef
- 1/2 cup onion, diced (about 2.5 oz)
- 2 cloves garlic, minced
- 4 slices bacon, cooked crisp and crumbled
- 1 1/2 cup cheese, shredded

Instructions:

TO CRUST:

Preheat the oven to 425 ° C

Combine the cream and mozzarella cheese in a large safe microwave mixing bowl. 1 Minute Microwave. Remove it from microwave, then mix to blend. Return to the microwave for another one minute.

Add garlic powder, milk, Italian seasoning, almond flour, onion powder, maritime, black pepper, and sea salt to mixing cup. Mix until well-incorporated ingredients are all in. (It'll be hard and stiff to mix.)

Line a 12-inch parchment-papered pizza pan. Break the "dough" into a thin sheet then coat the pizza plate. If the dough is unworkable or too stingy, just place it back in the microwave to soften for 1 minute.

Bake for 10-12 minutes or until its golden brown, on the middle rack. Watch it to ensure it's not bubbling up. If it is required, using a toothpick to blow up some bubbles.

FOR TOPPING:

Mix yellow mustard with a low carbohydrates pizza sauce and put it on the side. Inside a saute pan, mix the ground beef, garlic, and onion on medium heat.

Saute until ground beef is soft and onions are cooked through. Drain some excess oil.

PLACING IT TOGETHER:

Pour pizza sauce uniformly over the top of the pie.

Top with one even cheese layer

Pile the mixture on the ground beef.

Top it with slices of pickles and crumbled bacon.

Lower the heat to 350 °

Bake it for another 10 minutes.

Nutrition:

Serving Size: 1 slice

Per Serving – 1 Slice

Total Carbs – 8.5 Fiber – 2g

Calories – 400 Protein – 21g Fat – 20g

Net Carbs – 6.5

4.21 Beef and Chorizo Low Carb Empanadas

Yield= 12 empanadas

Ingredients:

FOR FILLING:

8 green olives, chopped

8 ounces pork chorizo

8 ounces ground beef

1/2 cup diced onion

2 tablespoons tomato paste

2 cloves garlic, minced

Sea salt and black pepper, to taste

3 green onions, chopped

2 hardboiled eggs, chopped

FOR DOUGH:

3 tablespoons cream cheese

1/2 teaspoon black pepper

1 1/2 cups mozzarella cheese, shredded

3/4 cup almond flour

1 teaspoon garlic powder

1 large egg

1 teaspoon onion powder

1 teaspoon of sea salt

1 teaspoon Italian seasoning

Instructions:

FOR FILLING:

Add the ground beef, onion, garlic, pepper, pork chorizo, and sea salt in a large skillet. Sauté on medium flame until cooking is done through the meat. Drain the excess grease and then mix in the paste for tomatoes. Stir water for another five minutes.

Transfer the mixture to the bowl and mix in the eggs, olives, and green onions. Put it aside

FOR DOUGH:

Add cream cheese and mozzarella cheese in a large blending bowl. 1 Minute Microwave. Stir it to combine and add one extra minute to microwave.

Mix in egg, almond flour, garlic powder, Italian seasoning, onion powder, black pepper, and sea salt. Mix when all the components are blended properly.

BY COMBING BOTH:

Line 2 baking sheets with rim with a parchment or Silpat paper. Spread your dough out over one of the sheets in a flimsy even layer. Draw circles into your dough using the rim of a bowl. Place circles onto the other sheet of baking.

Ball up the dough again. Repeat until you've got 12 circles.

Oven preheat to 425 ° C

Spoon that meat mixture onto every circle. Fold the dough over the meat mound and tap the edges. Use a fork to tap the edges.

Bake twelve minutes or to brown before white.

Nutrition:

Per Serving = 2 Empanadas

Fat: 25 g, Calories: 344, Carbs: 7.5 net grams, Protein: 26 g, Net Carbs: 6.5, Fiber: 1 g

4.22 Fat Head Waffle Pepperoni Pizza Dippers

Yield: 4 servings Cooking Time=10 minutes, Prep Time=10 minutes, Total Time=20 minutes,

INGREDIENTS:

- 1 large egg
- 1 teaspoon garlic powder
- 3/4 cup blanched almond flour
- 3 tablespoons cream cheese

- 1/2 teaspoon dried oregano
- 1 teaspoon onion powder
- 1/2 teaspoon black pepper
- 1 1/2 cup mozzarella cheese, shredded
- 1 teaspoon Italian seasoning
- ¼ cup pizza sauce with extra for dipping
- 1/4 cup shredded mozzarella cheese
- 12 slices pepperoni

Instructions:

Pre-heat the waffle iron

Combine the cream and mozzarella cheese in a broad safe microwave mixing dish. 1 Minute Microwave. Remove from microwave, and combine to stir. Microwave it for another 1 minute.

Add egg, Italian seasoning, almond flour, onion powder, black pepper, and garlic powder to mixing bowl. Mix all the ingredients until they are properly uncooperative. If your dough becomes unworkable or too sticky, then water your hands and place your dough on a parchment paper piece and divide it into 2 balls of the same size.

Top with two spoonfuls of pizza sauce and then 6 pepperoni slices. Cover the lid. Cook until the heating of dough is finished, and the sides are crispy and soft. Remove your pizza with two tablespoons of the mozzarella cheese & one-fourth teaspoon of oregano from waffle iron and top.

The exact process is repeated with another piece of the dough.

Then cut the completed waffles into 4ths and serve, for dipping, with additional pizza sauce.

Nutrition:

Net Carbohydrates per Serving= 3g

Serving Size=2 pieces, Fat: 14g, Calories: 362, Fiber: 2g, Carbohydrates: 5g, Protein: 10g

4.23 Keto Cinnamon Rolls

Yield: 8 servings Cooking Time: 20 minutes, Prep Time: 25 minutes, Total Time: 45 minutes,

Ingredients:

FOR DOUGH:

- 2 ounces cream cheese
- 1 1/2 cups low moisture, part-skim shredded mozzarella cheese
- 1 1/4 teaspoon baking powder
- 1 cup almond flour
- 1 tablespoon powdered erythritol
- 1 large egg
- 1/2 teaspoon pure vanilla extract

FOR FILLING:

- 1 1/2 tablespoons cinnamon
- 1/2 teaspoon maple extract
- 5 tablespoons butter, melted
- 1/4 cup brown sugar erythritol
- 1/2 cup chopped pecans

FOR GLAZE:

- 1/2 teaspoon maple extract
- 1 tablespoon powdered erythritol
- 1/3 cup heavy cream
- 1/2 teaspoon pure vanilla extract
- Pinch of the sea salt

Instructions:

MAKING DOUGH:

Pre - heat to 400 ° F on the burner. Fill a baking pan with light grease.

Combine the cream and mozzarella cheese for about 30 seconds at a time in your microwave-safe bowl & then microwave, before the cheese is molten sufficiently to blend.

Mix in your almond flour, milk, baking powder, erythritol, and vanilla extract until the cheeses have been melted and mixed. Mix until all of the items have been well incorporated and form a dough.

Spread out the dough between 2 parchment paper sheets then cool it for 15 minutes.

MAKING FILLING:

In a bowl, mix melted butter and extracts together, while the dough is cooling.

Brush over the dough the butter mixture and leave an approximately one-inch gap across the edges of the dough, then sprinkle the cinnamon, erythritol, and pecans in brown sugar over the top.

Use your parchment paper to enable rolling the dough, roll it tightly and cut it off carefully, and discard the unequal edges.

Slice the dough into eight even rolls using a sharp knife. (Wetting the knife may help to keep the dough from trying to stick to it, as you slice the rolls)

Place the rolls in the baking pan snuggly but not too close, because they need space to expand when cooking. Brush it with leftover maple butter and cover with parchment paper loosely over the sheet. Bake for eight minutes. Remove the paper from the

Parchment and bake for an extra 10 minutes.

DOWN THE GLAZE:

When they bake the cinnamon rolls, plan the glaze. In a shallow cup, insert the heavy cream, vanilla extract, erythritol, syrup extract, and salt and mix with a whisk. An electric mixer can also be used to whip this to make a thicker glaze that you can pipe over the cinnamon rolls, and once your cinnamon rolls have baked, make them cool for five minutes and after that drizzle over the top of the glaze.

Nutrition:

Net carbohydrates per serving (1 cinnamon roll) =3.2g

Serving Size: 1 cinnamon roll, Fat: 28.2g, Calories: 296, Carbohydrates: 5.1g, Protein: 8.7g Fiber: 1.9g,

4.24 Fried Cabbage with Kielbasa (Low Carb, Gluten-Free)

Yield: 6 Servings Cooking Time: 20 minutes, Prep Time: 10 minutes, Total Time: 30 minutes.

Ingredients:

- 1 cup onion, diced (about 4 oz)
- 6 tbsp butter
- 4 cloves garlic, minced
- 14 oz kielbasa, thinly sliced
- 1 tsp crushed red pepper flakes, optional
- 2 tbsp red wine vinegar
- Large head green cabbage, cored and sliced
- Sea salt and pepper, to taste
- 1 tsp paprika
- 1/4 cup Italian flat-leaf parsley, rough chopped

Instructions:

Melt 3 tablespoons of butter into a large skillet on medium heat. Add some garlic and onion to the saucepan. Sauté it until garlic is fragrant and onion is brownish.

Add the red wine vinegar in the saucepan and mix it with garlic and onions.

Add the sliced kielbasa into the saucepan and sauté till browned.

Then add the remaining butter, chicken powder, salt, paprika, and pepper. Mix all the ingredients and coat the cob with seasoning and butter.

Saute it until wilted as well as slightly browned on cabbage.

Before serving, top off with red crushed pepper flakes and fresh parsley.

Nutrition:

Per serving protein – 6g Net Carbs – 9.5 Calories – 370 Fat – 29g 5 Fiber – 7g Total Carbs – 16

4.25 Pork Egg Roll in a Bowl (Keto, Paleo, Whole30)

If you don't care to keep this Whole30 compliant or paleo, feel free to replace coconut aminos with soy sauce. You can use tamari, as well.

Yield: 6 Servings Cooking Time: 25 minutes, Prep Time: 5 minutes, Total Time: 30 minutes,

Ingredients:

- 3 cloves garlic, minced
- 2 tablespoons sesame oil
- 1/2 cup onion, diced
- 1-pound ground pork
- 5 green onions, cut (both green and white parts)
- 1/2 teaspoon grounded ginger
- 2 tablespoons toasted sesame seeds
- 1 tablespoon garlic or sriracha chili sauce, to taste
- Sea salt and black pepper, to taste
- 14-ounce bag of coleslaw mix

- 1 tablespoon unseasoned rice vinegar
- 3 tbsp. Coconut Aminos or soy sauce (gluten-free)

Instructions:

In a wide skillet, boil up sesame oil on medium-high flame.

Add your white parts of green onions with garlic and onion. Sauté it until garlic is fragranced, and onion is transparent.

Add the powdered pork, powdered ginger, black pepper, sea salt, and Sriracha. Saute before the bacon is thoroughly cooked.

Add the mixture of coleslaw, coconut aminos, and vinegar for rice wine. You have to Saute till coleslaw is complete.

Nutrition:

Carbohydrates per serving=5.5g net

Fat: 20g, Calories: 297, Carbohydrates: 7g, Protein: 20g Fiber: 1.5g,

4.26 Cabbage Noodle Tuna Casserole (Low Carb, Gluten-Free)

Yield: Makes 8 servings Cooking Time: 30 minutes, Prep Time: 15 minutes, Total Time: 45 minutes,

Ingredients:

- 2 tbsp grass-fed butter
- 2 tbsp olive oil
- 1/2 cup frozen peas
- Medium head green cabbage (about 1 1/2 lbs.), cut into large shreds
- 3 ribs celery, chopped
- 1 cup onion, chopped
- 2 cloves garlic, minced
- 2 tsp dried dill

- Sea salt and black pepper, to taste
- 2 tsp dry mustard powder
- Juice of 1 lemon
- 2 tbsp lemon zest
- 1 1/2 cup heavy cream
- 3 – 5oz cans albacore tuna, drained
- 1 1/4 cup Parmesan cheese

Instructions:

In an extra-large, ovenproof skillet, heat the butter and olive oil over medium heat.

Add the onion, cabbage, sea salt, celery, black pepper, and garlic to the saucepan once heated.

Drizzle until vegetables are tender for about ten minutes.

Mix the dill with the lemon zest, mustard powder, and lemon juice together.

In the pan, pour your heavy cream as well as 1 cup of Parmesan cheese. Mix in and continue to stir until the cheese melts and combines with heavy cream. Lower the flame to medium-low, and allow it to simmer to thicken the sauce.

Stir in your tuna and peas after the sauce has begun thickening.

Spread the rest of the Parmesan on the top of the platter and move to the oven and then broil on high for about 3 to 5 minutes or until a brownish golden crust has been formed by the Parmesan on the top.

Nutrition:

Carbohydrates per serving=7g net

Fat: 28g, Calories: 377, Carbohydrates: 10g, Protein: 23.5g Fiber: 3g,

4.27 Cheesy Sausage and Cabbage Casserole

Yield: 8 Servings Cooking Time: 35 minutes, Prep Time: 15 minutes, Total Time: 50 minutes,

Ingredients:

- 2 tbsp grass-fed butter
- 2 tbsp olive oil
- 1 1/2 cups mozzarella cheese, shredded
- Medium head green cabbage cored quartered and sliced
- 1 cup onion, diced
- 4 cloves garlic, minced
- 1 yellow bell pepper, chopped
- Sea salt and black pepper, to taste
- 1 1/2 cup crushed tomatoes
- 14.5 oz can dice tomatoes
- 14 oz smoked sausage, halved and sliced into half-moons
- 1/4 cup Italian flat-leaf parsley, rough chopped

Instructions:

Preheat the oven to 400 ° C

In a big skillet, heat up butter and olive oil on medium heat.

Then add cabbage, onion garlic, bell pepper, black pepper, and sea salt once your butter has been melted as well as the pan has been heated. Saute until vegetable is tender, and wilting the cabbage — approximately ten minutes.

Mix together in sliced tomatoes, roasted tomatoes, plus the smoked sausages. Saute it on for ten minutes.

Move to a large saucepan, top with the cheese, and then bake it for 15 minutes. Before the serving, top it with parsley.

Nutrition:

Carbohydrates per serving=8g net

Fat: 25g, Calories: 333, Carbohydrates: 11.75g, Protein: 15.5g Fiber: 3.75g,

---

4.28 Oven Roasted Cabbage Wedges

Yield: 6 Servings Cooking Time: 45 minutes, Prep Time: 15 minutes, Total Time: 1 hour,

Ingredients:

- ¼ teaspoon black pepper
- ¼ Cup Olive Oil
- 1 Head Green Cabbage
- 1 ½ teaspoon garlic salt
- 1 teaspoon fennel seeds
- 1 teaspoon onion powder

Instructions:

Preheat to 400 ° F on the oven. Line a half-sheet pan with a baking mat of silicone, and otherwise parchment paper.

Split the cabbage from head to toe in 1 "strips. (Stem underneath)

Lines slice onto the baking sheet in a single layer. Brush with a generous olive oil coating to each wedge.

Combine the garlic oil, fennel seed, onion powder, and black pepper in a small bowl. Sprinkle over each wedge for seasoning.

Bake for 45 minutes – turning nearly halfway through.

Nutrition:

Per Serving =1 Slice, Calories – 120, Net Carbs – 5g, protein – 2g, Total Carbs – 9g, Fiber – 4g, Fat – 9g

Serving Size=1 Slice

4.29 Low Carb Cauliflower Hash Browns

Fritters of cauliflower are very easy to make and also very versatile-think base, side, or snack. They make browns with the finest low carb hash.

Servings: 12, Course: Side Dish, Prep Time: 15 minutes, Cook Time: 20 minutes, Cuisine: Vegetarian, Total Time: 35 minutes, Calories: 69kcal

Ingredients:

- Cauliflower
- 1 teaspoon salt
- Fritters
- 1/2 cup almond flour
- 1-pound raw cauliflower, grated
- 1/2 cup grated Parmesan cheese
- 3 ounces onion chopped
- 4 large eggs
- 1/2 teaspoon baking powder
- 1 1/2 teaspoons lemon pepper

Instructions:

Scrape the cauliflower in a colander, then sprinkle the salt and mix well with your hands. Let the cauliflower rest for about ten minutes.

Meanwhile, the onions are chopped and placed in a medium bowl. Then squeeze the water out from the cauliflower with clean hands, and put the cauliflower with the onions in the medium bowl. Add baking powder, flour, cheese, and seasoning to the almond. Mix carefully. Add the three eggs, then mix until they are incorporated.

Skillet technique: Place medium heat on a frying pan or skillet. Add 1 table cubit of oil when hot. Scoop your cauliflower fritter batter out and place it into the hot skillet using a measuring cup of 1/4th. Softly move a spatula down to create a smooth pancake—Cook 3 minutes to each side. Drain on towels made from cotton. Do not flip the fritter until it is well cooked to the bottom.

Method Oven: Preheat your oven to 400 degrees F. Line 2 parchment cookie sheets. Measure 1/4th cup of batter for each squander and flatten into a circle. Bake for 10-12 minutes, then turn the other side down and bake for another 10-12 minutes.

Store it in the fridge. Reheat over medium heat in a dry skillet to make it crisp again.

Nutrition Facts:

Low Carb Cauliflower Hash Browns

Amount per Serving

Calories 69Calories from Fat 36

% Daily Value*

Carbohydrates 4g 1%

Fiber 1g 4%

Protein 5g 10%

Fat 4g 6%

Nutrition:

Fiber: 1g | Carbohydrates: 4g | Protein: 5g | Calories: 69kcal | Fat: 4g

Chapter 5: Sweet Recipes for Keto Breakfast

This chapter will introduce you with the vast and basic recipes containing a variety of ingredients regarding Keto desserts. These Dessert recipes are exclusively for those who are on this diet or going for healthy and clean food.

5.1 Keto Chocolate Frosty

Prep time: 10 minutes

Total time: 10 minutes

Yield: 4 servings

Ingredients:

- 1 cup heavy whipping cream
- 1 teaspoon vanilla extract
- 2 tablespoons unsweetened cocoa powder
- 1 tablespoon almond butter
- 1/2 teaspoon liquid stevia sweetener

Instructions:

Use the egg beaters to mix all items together until peaks form, which will be stiff.

Place it in the refrigerator for 30-60 minutes until it is frozen barely.

Then place your frosty in a plastic freezer container, cut one of the corners, and pipe into different tiny cups.

Nutritional Information:

Serving Size: 1 Frosty, Yield: 4 servings

Amount per Serving: Calories: 241, Total Fat: 25g, Fiber: 1g, Total Carbohydrates: 4g, Net Carbohydrates: 3g, Protein: 3g

5.2 Low-Carb Orange Julius:

Prep time: 5 minutes

Yield: 2 servings

Total time: 5 minutes

This simple to create a recipe for Orange Julius is creamy, frothy, and with a fresh orange taste.

Ingredients:

- 2/3 cup heavy whipping cream

- 3 tablespoons erythritol, confectioners

- 1 1/2 teaspoons pure orange extract

- Food coloring (optional for orange color)

- 2 tablespoons cream cheese

- Orange slice (optional for garnish)

- 1 1/2 teaspoons lemon juice

Instructions:

Stir in heavy cream to combine. (You have to prefer using a personal-sized, lightweight blender). Blend for around a minute before your cream has churned into a dense whipped cream.

Add cream cheese, pure orange extract, erythritol, lemon juice, (if desired) food coloring, and broken ice. (You can use broken ice over ice cubes allows the shake to easily fall together). Blend until smooth and even, around a minute.

Pour into one or two small containers. Where desired, garnish it with an orange slice. Love it!

Recipe notes:

Freeze leftovers to eat later in a freezer-safe / microwave-safe bag. When able, either melt at room temperature or put in the microwave for 30-45 seconds, then defrost at high heat. Frozen leftovers remind you of sherbet in raspberry. It will be yum.

Also, note that the nutritional information does not include a selectable orange slice for garnish. One orange slice possesses about 1.5 g of net carbs.

Nutritional information:

Serving Size: 1 cup, Yield: 2 servings

Amount per Serving: Calories: 325, Protein: 3g, Net Carbohydrates: 2.5g, Fiber: 0g, Total Carbohydrates: 16g, Sugar Alcohols: 13.5g, Total Fat: 34g

5.3 Keto Sugar-Free Krispy Kreme Doughnuts

Prep time: 30 minutes

Cook time: 18 minutes

Total time: 48 minutes

Humid, fuzzy, and gentle. 100 percent yummy. You might want to increase the amounts because they are going to vanish soon.

Ingredients:

For the doughnuts:

- 2 large eggs
- 80g full fat cream cheese
- 40g erythritol
- ½ tsp pure stevia powder
- 20g unsalted butter
- 30g vanilla whey protein powder

- 10g fine psyllium husk powder

- Pinch of fine Himalayan pink salt

- 2 tsp baking powder

- 2 tsp apple cider vinegar (ACV)

For the optional frosting (various choices):

- 120g mascarpone

- 15g Sukrin icing sugar

- A few drops vanilla extract

- Pitaya powder for pink topping

- Maqui powder for lilac topping

- Unsweetened dark chocolate, min 85%

Instructions:

For creating the Doughnuts:

Preheat oven to fan 150 ° C (static at 170 ° C).

Whisk the cream cheese, eggs, salt, and sweeteners together.

Melt butter and cool it a bit, then mix it into the mixture of eggs.

To obtain an even batter, combine whey, baking powder, psyllium, and ACV before adding it to the moist mix and hand whisk it all.

In your doughnut molds, scoop the (runny) batter so that it is divided evenly and equally.

Bake for Eighteen minutes, then turn off the oven, and open the door and leave for another 5 minutes before removing.

Let the doughnuts fully cool down, then erase them from their moldings.

To have the frosting done:

Beat the mascarpone until fluffy, then apply the icing sugar and thoroughly blend.

Now you have choices that you can either apply a couple of vanilla extract drops or melt dark chocolate (you will need 40 g), or 1 tsp maqui (lilac), or 1 tsp pitaya (pink).

Using a thin, lightweight cake-decorating spatula to distribute the frosting all over, bar the undersides.

Recipe notes:

Macros mentioned above are for one simple doughnut, although they may be 'customized' in several ways.

Macros for each doughnut including mascarpone frosting, add:

Vanilla: Kcal 66; C 0.4g; P 0.6g, F 7g.

Pitaya/Maqui: Kcals 70; P 0.6g, F 7g; C 0.5g.

Chocolate: Kcals 74; C 0.7g; F 7.5g; P 1g.

Nutrition:

Yield: 8

Calories: 86

Cuisine: Ketogenic. Sugar-Free. Grain-Free. LCHF. Low Carb. Gluten-Free.

Serving: 1

Fat: 7g

Protein: 4g

Recipe type: Desserts

Net Carbs: 1.3g

5.4 Flourless Keto Chewy Double Chocolate Chip Cookies

Prep Time: 10 minutes, Time required: 22 minutes, Cook Time: 12 minutes,

Yield: 18

Ingredients:

- 1 cup natural creamy almond butter
- 1 1/2 teaspoons pure vanilla extract
- 2 tablespoons unsweetened cocoa powder
- 2/3 cup powdered monk fruit
- 2 tablespoons peanut butter powder
- 1 tablespoon melted salted butter
- 2 large eggs
- 2 tablespoons water
- 1/4 cup sugar-free chocolate chips
- 1 teaspoon baking soda

Instructions:

Preheat, the oven up to 350 ° F. Cover your rimmed baking sheet with a baking mat of silicone or parchment paper.

Combine the chocolate powder, peanut butter paste, almond butter, monk fruit, bacon, milk, sugar, baking soda, and vanilla extract into a large mixing cup. Blend until all components are well mixed, utilizing an electronic hand mixer. It's going to be a very thick dough. Chocolate chips fold in. Shape the cookie dough into 1 1/2 "to 2" balls. To yield more cookies, you can make them smaller.

Layer the balls of cookie dough on the lined baking dish. Bake for 8 to 11 minutes (at 8 minutes, start checking on them). To encourage the cookies to cool before consuming, remove your baking sheet from the microwave and put it on a cooling rack.

Nutrition:

Serving Size: 1 cookie, Fat: 10g, Protein: 4g, Carbohydrates: 3.8g, Calories: 115, Fiber: 2.4g,

5.5 Mini Keto Blueberry Cheesecakes

Prep Time: 10 minutes, Time required: 40 minutes, Cook Time: 30 minutes, Yield: 12 mini cheesecakes

Ingredients:

FOR THE CRUST

- 1 cup almond flour
- 1/4 cup salted butter, melted
- 1 tbsp golden monk fruit

FOR THE FILLING

- 16 oz cream cheese, room temperature
- 2 tsp lemon extract
- 1/2 cup granular monk fruit
- 2 large pastured eggs
- 1 tsp vanilla extract

FOR THE TOPPING

- 1 cup frozen blueberries

Instructions:

Use a standard silicone muffin pan or line up a regular muffin pan by using muffin liners.

The brown sugar erythritol and the almond flour are combined in a medium mixing bowl. Add the melted butter to your bowl and then mix until it coats the almond flour and is the wet sand texture. In the muffin pan, divide the mixture uniformly among the 12 wells. Use one spoon to press the mixture evenly down into each muffin liner's bottom.

Bake for 5 minutes at the crusts.

Using a hand brush, pound the cream cheese in a large mixing bowl until they become soft.

Add the eggs, vanilla extract, lemon extract, and Swerve and mix until all the ingredients are smooth and well combined. To scrape the sides using a rubber spatula and mix in.

In the muffin pan, evenly divide the mixture of cheesecake among all 12 wells. Put this on top of a baking sheet when using a silicone muffin pan.

Bake till the cheesecakes are set for 25 -30 minutes. They are always going to be a bit jiggly in the middle.

Enable for 20 minutes to cool off on the oven.

Then heat up a small saucepan over the medium flame while your cheesecakes are cooling, and add the blueberries. Give the blueberries 15 minutes to simmer. Slightly mash them to release their juices and thicken the juices. Equally, divide blueberries among the cheesecakes.

Then chill in before serving for up to 24 hours.

Nutrition:

4.75g net carbs per serving

Serving Size: 1 mini cheesecake, Fat: 21g, Protein: 5.5g, Calories: 233, Fiber: 1.75g, Carbohydrates: 6.5g.

5.6 Low Carb Flourless Chocolate Peanut Butter Cake

Yield=1 Serving

Components:

- 2 tbsp unsweetened organic cocoa powder
- 1 tsp salted butter
- 1/2 tsp vanilla extract
- 1 large pastured egg
- 2 tbsp. erythritol or Swerve Sweetener
- 1 tablespoon heavy cream
- 1/4 tablespoon baking powder
- 1 tablespoon peanut butter

Directions:

Combine chocolate powder, baking powder, and sweetener into a tiny mixing cup. Fork stir to mix and mash some clumps of baking powder.

Combine the heavy cream, vanilla extract, and egg in a single, shallow mixing pot. Whisk to blend. Pour the moist ingredients into dry. Blend once fully blended into the materials. Melt your butter in the small bowl or a ramekin and swirl then for coating.

Pour the batter into ramekin butter.

1 min and some seconds Microwave.

In your microwave, melt peanut butter and then drizzle over the top of the meal.

Nutrition:

Per serving- Protein= 10 g | Calories= 246 | Net Carbohydrates= 5 g | Fat=19 g

5.7 Low Carb Chocolate Mason Jar Ice Cream

Optional sugar-free chocolate chips do not include in nutritional information.

Prep Time: 8 minutes, Yield: 2 cups (4 Servings), Total Time: 8 minutes.

Ingredients:

- 2 tablespoons sugar-free chocolate chips, optional
- 1 cup heavy cream
- 2 tablespoons granular monk fruit
- 1 tablespoon unsweetened cocoa powder
- 2 tablespoons granular monk fruit
- 1 teaspoon pure vanilla extract

Instructions:

Mix the ingredients in a mason jar with a wide mouth. Screw the lid on, then shake for 5 minutes. The fluid in the side is supposed to become twice in volume while filling Mason jar.

Then freeze for up to 24 hours.

Scoop and have fun.

Nutrition:

2.25g net carbs per serving

Serving Size: 1/2 cup, Fat: 22g, Protein: 1g, Calories: 206.

5.8 Paleo Mixed Berry Coconut Creamsicles (Low Carb Popsicles)

Paleo Coconut Mixed Berry Creamsicles-Low Carbohydrates Popsicles. You can now have all of the childhood flavors in a healthier version.

Yield=10 Popsicles

Ingredients:

- 1 1/2 cups frozen mixed berries
- 1 cup of water
- 3 tbsp. erythritol, more to taste
- 1 tbsp lemon juice
- 1 tsp vanilla extract
- 1 1/2 cups coconut milk
- 1 tsp vanilla bean paste

Instructions:

Combine the mixed berries, water, and the lemon juice in the medium saucepan. Bring on medium to high heat to a bowl. Reduce the heat when it starts to boil and let it boil till your berries pop up and start releasing their juices. By using a fork mash in the liquid the berries in.

Combine the vanilla extract, coconut milk, erythritol, and bean paste in another saucepan. Whisk together. Let it boil and after that, reduce to low heat and allow it to simmer. Stirring often, let your mixture simmer till it begins to thicken even a little bit.

Combine all saucepans and then whisk material before all components are fully absorbed. Let's get cool.

Mix until the mixture is poured in the Popsicle molds one last time.

Fill the pot, attach the sticks to the Popsicle, and freeze to the firm.

Nutrition:

2.3g net carbohydrates per serving

Serving Size: 1 Popsicle, Fat: 0.7g, Calories: 21, Fiber: 1.1g, Carbohydrates: 3.4g,

5.9 Low Carb Chocolate Peanut Butter Bars

Yield: 16 bars Cook Time: 20 minutes, Prep Time: 10 minutes, Total Time: 30 minutes.

Ingredients:

- 1 large egg
- 4 oz cream cheese, softened
- 1 tsp vanilla extract
- 2 cups almond flour
- 1/2 cup heavy cream
- 1/2 cup natural chunky peanut butter
- 3 tbsp granular monk fruit, more if you like it sweeter
- 1/2 cup sugar-free chocolate chips

Instructions:

Preheat the oven to 350 o.

Using the hand mixer, combine cream cheese and the egg in a broad mixing bowl until it becomes creamy.

Add the almond flour, heavy cream, peanut butter, vanilla extract, and sweetener to the mixing pot. Mix when all the components are blended properly.

Insert chocolate chips onto the mixture, use the rubber spatula.

Move the mixture to a baking pan 88 non-stick.

Bake for another 20 minutes.

Nutrition Facts

Easy No-Bake Peanut Butter Bars

Amount Per serving (1 bar)

Calories 216Calories from Fat 168

% Daily Value

Fat 18.7g29%

Carbohydrates 7.2g2%

Fiber 2.9g12%

Protein 5.6g11%

5.10 Keto Brownie Ice Cream

Rich and tasty, this Ice Cream Keto Brownie is the great summer delight. It's so nice you won't know it's low in carb and it's gluten-free.

Yield: 8 servings, Category: Dessert Cook Time: 30 minutes, Prep Time: 3 hours, Total Time: 3 hours 30 minutes.

Ingredients:

- 3.5 ounces sugar-free chocolate chips (100g)
- 1 3/4 cup heavy cream, divided
- 1/3 cup powdered monk fruit
- 4 Fudgy Double Chocolate Keto Brownies
- 1/2 teaspoon pure vanilla extract
- 3 large egg yolks, room temperature

- 1 tablespoon smooth almond butter

Instructions:

Heat one cup of heavy cream over low heat in a saucepan. Add chocolate chips to your pan and stir regularly and heat till the chocolate has melted completely.

Beat egg yolks and monk fruit together, using your electric mixer until thick and pale.

Add egg mixture to the refrigerated chocolate and then mix together. Return your pan to low flame and swirl continuously for around 1 minute before it thickens. Don't allow your mixture to get into a bubble, or it breaks. Take the mixture into a bowl and allow it to cool.

Whip the rest of the three fourth cup of your heavy cream using your electric mixer until thick, steep peaks form. Fold the chocolate mixture that is cooled down into whipped cream, along with almond extract and almond butter. If your mixture becomes too thick, add 2 to 3 tablespoons of unflavored almond milk to thin out.

Pour ice cream mixture in an ice cream maker and proceed according to instructions from the manufacturers. This may take 15-45 minutes, based on which ice cream maker is used.

When the ice cream has been done, transfer it into a big container that is freezable just as the pictured loaf pan. Cover in brownie pieces and then freeze for 1-2 hours, or before you achieve the perfect consistency.

When you take the ice cream out from the fridge, only until you eat it, encourage it to rest on the counter.

Nutrition:

Net carbohydrates per serving=6.3g

Fat: 32.5g, Calories: 350, Fiber: 2.5g, Carbohydrates: 8.8g, Protein: 6g

5.11 Low Carb Blueberry Muffins

Yield=6 Muffins

Ingredients:

CREAM WITH:

- 4 tablespoons (2 oz) cream cheese, very soft
- 1/2 teaspoon of vanilla
- ½ stick (2 oz) butter, very soft

DRY INGREDIENTS

- ¼ cup granular monk fruit
- ½ cup coconut flour
- 1 teaspoon baking powder
- 1/16 teaspoon cinnamon
- 1/8 teaspoon of xanthan gum
- 1/4 teaspoon salt

WET INGREDIENTS:

- 1/4 cup of heavy cream
- 3 large eggs (cold)

ADD LAST:

- 2 teaspoons granular monk fruit
- 1/3 cup of fresh blueberries

Instructions:

PREPARATION:

Preheat the oven to 350 degrees C. Place the oven rack in the bottom 3rd of the oven. Cover a six-cup muffin tray with liner ink. For a smaller tub, put all dry ingredients simultaneously, and sweep together to mix and separate any lumps if present.

COMBINE:

Cream the cream, vanilla, and cheese, butter together in a medium bowl until fluffy and light. In your butter mixture, add one egg and then beat until your mixture is fluffy and light (it can separate and break, it's ok). Add one-third of dry ingredients. Blend until thoroughly combined, maintaining the sweet, fluffy feel intact. Keep in mind that during this process that you want a fluffy and light texture, almost like a mousse.

Add an egg and then beat until the mix is full and your batter becomes fluffy. Then add half of your dry ingredients leftover and beat again. Add one last potato and beating until thoroughly added, and the rest of your dry ingredients follow. Once again, end by adding heavy cream. Beat until batter is dense but fluffy and light.

Fold in blueberries

FILLING OF THE MUFFIN TIN:

Spoon the dense batter in a zip-lock plastic bag and then snip off the corner, making around a 3/4 "opening. Put your sliced corner in the muffin liner. Push the batter in a large, fat pile, filling muffin liner of about three fourth completely. Repeat this for each liner of muffins, adding any leftover batter to the ones that need more. Knock your finger over any peaks. Sprinkle around 1/4 teaspoon of the monk fruit over every muffin to prevent the burning as well as provide a fine look to the muffins.

BAKE:

Place your muffins in the microwave. Turn your oven for five minutes, until 400 ° degrees. Switch your oven to 350 °, then for another 25 minutes, bake your blueberry muffins. m When you press a finger slightly, they're ready if they see are firm, but they still seem moist a little and then remove them from your oven and then let it cool for five mins, before removing gently from your pan and putting it on the cooling rack.

Nutrition:

4g net carbohydrates per serving

Serving Size: 1 Muffin, Fat: 25g, Calories: 273, Carbohydrates: 7g, Protein: 5g, Fiber: 3g.

5.12 Keto Chewy Chocolate and Peanut Butter Bacon Cookies

Yield= 12 Cookies

Ingredients:

- 1 cup of chunky peanut butter
- 1 tsp baking soda
- 6 slices bacon, cooked crisp and crumbled
- 1 cup granular sweetener
- 1/2 cup unsweetened cocoa powder that is organic
- 1 large egg
- 1 1/2 tablespoon vanilla extract

Instructions:

Cook the bacon, crumble and put aside until crisp.

Oven preheat to 350 ° C

Combine sweetener, peanut butter, and egg in one big mixing pot. Blend before both components fall together. Put the gloves on and do this with your hands. There was rich peanut butter, and that just made things better.

Add some cocoa powder, baking soda, and vanilla extract to the mixture. Mix till all the ingredients have mixed well.

Throw over crumbled bacon.

Using a parchment paper or Silpat, cover the baking dish.

Shape dough in twelve balls of equal measure, place on a liner. Flatten only a little bit.

 Bake inside ten mins. Remove from the oven and put the baking sheet onto a refrigerating rack. Unless you don't encourage the cookies to cool down completely, they'll break in pieces.

Nutritional facts:

Serving Size=one Cookie

5.13 Low Carb Chocolate Mocha Cupcakes

Each cupcake contains just less than 5 net carbs (that depend on the sugar-free chocolate chip brand used)

Yield=Makes 9 Cupcakes

Ingredients:

- 1/4 cup coconut flour
- 1 cup almond flour
- 1/4 cup organic cocoa powder
- 2 teaspoons aluminum-free baking powder
- 1/4 cup granular erythritol
- 3 large eggs

- 2 teaspoon coffee extract

- 1/2 cup coconut milk

- 1 teaspoon pure vanilla extract

- 1/4 cup sugar-free chocolate chips

- 1/4 cup salted grass-fed butter, melted

Instructions:

Using a silicone muffin tray or fill a muffin box with the paper muffin cups to preheat the oven to 350 °.

Add the almond meal, coconut flour, Swerve, chocolate powder, and baking powder to a large mixing pot. Combine whisk to ensure that baking powder is properly mixed and is not clumped.

Beat the eggs in a separate bowl. Mix then coffee extract, coconut milk, vanilla extract, and butter melted.

Place your wet ingredients in your dry ingredients and combine them when pouring. Mix well until combined.

Then stir in some chocolate chips and save some on top of cupcakes to sprinkle with.

A mixture of the spoon into packed muffin cups. Cover of extra chocolate chips and bake for twenty mins or until strong on tops. Allow cupcakes, on the top of the cooling rack, to cool in the tin.

Nutrition:

Serving Size=1 Cupcake

5.14 Keto Strawberry Cheesecake Ice Cream

This Strawberry Ice Cream Cheesecake keto is a true champion. It is creamy, sugar-free, and fruity. Full of keto-friendly fats, this is a frozen chubby bomb treat you're going to want to make over and over again.

Yield: 10 servings Cook Time: 30 minutes, Prep Time: 120 minutes, Total Time: 2 hours 30 minutes,

Ingredients:

FOR THE CRUMB TOPPING:

- 3 tablespoons whey protein
- 3/4 cup blanched almond flour
- 2 tablespoons powdered monk fruit
- 1 tablespoon unsweetened almond milk
- 1 tablespoon, plus 2 teaspoons butter
- 1/2 teaspoon pure vanilla extract
- 5 to 10 drops liquid stevia
- 1/8 teaspoon sea salt

FOR THE ICE CREAM:

- 1/2 cup powdered monk fruit
- 3/4 cup quartered strawberries
- 1/2 teaspoon xanthan gum
- 2 large egg yolks, room temperature
- 1/2 cup creme fraiche
- 1 cup mascarpone cheese, room temperature
- 1 1/2 cups heavy cream
- 1 1/2 teaspoons pure vanilla extract
- 1/2 cup unsweetened almond milk

Instructions:

FOR THE CRUMB TOPPING:

Spread almond flour over a baking sheet, and bake at 400 ° F for 5 minutes.

In a cup, place the whey protein, butter, toasted almond flour, monk fruit, almond milk, salt, vanilla extract, and stevia and combine until well mixed. Create pieces using your fingers by squeezing parts of the flour. Chill in the fridge for 30 minutes.

FOR THE ICE CREAM:

Puree all the strawberries utilizing a food processor or high-powered blender, then put aside.

Beat the egg yolks and monk fruit together with the electric mixer, until light and very well mixed.

Add the mascarpone and then cook the cream then beat until it is smooth.

Heavy cream, vanilla extract, almond milk, and xanthan gum will be included. Taste, and if necessary, apply more sweeteners to it.

Load your ice cream mixture in an ice cream machine and cycle according to directions from the manufacturers. It can take 30-90 mins depending on what ice cream machine is using.

If the ice cream has been finished, move it to a freezable tub, much like the pictured loaf tray. Fold the crumb mixture in ¾ and then run around each of the strawberries.

Then drizzle the remaining strawberry puree at the top and brush over the remainder of the crumb mixture. Put 1 to 2 hours in the freezer, and require positioning.

After the ice cream is withdrawn from the fridge, let it rest on the counter to melt only marginally before eating it.

Nutrition:

Fat: 38g, Calories: 383, Fiber: 1.3g, Carbohydrates: 4.6g, Protein: 6.3g

5.15 Keto Key Lime Pie Jars

Total Time: 15 minutes, Time required: 15 minutes, Yield: 4 servings

Ingredients:

CRUMB LAYER:

- 1/3 cup ground pecans
- 1/3 cup ground almonds
- 1 tablespoon powdered erythritol
- Pinch of sea salt
- 1 vanilla bean pod, scraped or 1/2 teaspoon pure vanilla extract
- 1 tablespoon butter or coconut oil, melted

FILLING:

- 3/4 cup mascarpone cheese
- 1 large avocado, peeled and pitted
- Juice of 2 limes
- 1/4 cup heavy whipping cream
- 1 tablespoon butter or coconut oil, melted
- 1/4 cup powdered erythritol
- Zest of 1 lime

Instructions:

CRUMB LAYER:

Combine in a broad mixing bowl, nuts, pecans, butter, cinnamon, erythritol, and oil together. Mix all ingredients until they are properly mixed

FILLING:

The avocado, heavy cream, mascarpone, powdered erythritol, lime zest, butter, and lime juice are combined in another mixing bowl. Beat the liquids with a hand mixer until the paste is smooth and doesn't have any clear clumps.

Then divide the mixture of crumbs equally across 4 bottles. Spoon key lime mixture over the crumb layer and then evenly divide it among your 4 jars. Cover with some crumb's leftover.

Until eating, cool down for 30 to 60 mins.

Nutrition:

NET CARBS PER SERVING=5.3g

Carbohydrates: 10.5g, Fat: 46g, Protein: 6.6g, Fiber: 5.2g.

Chapter 6: Keto Salads, Appetizers, and Low Carb Smoothies

This chapter will let you learn about the recipes that are low in carbs as well as gluten-free. All of the basic recipes for Keto salads, dressings, and appetizers, along with their particular ingredients, are discussed in detail and depth in this chapter. It will guide you to the best.

6.1 Creamy Low-Carb Coleslaw

Yield: 6 servings

Prep time: 5 minutes

Total time: 5 minutes

This zesty, creamy coleslaw is a favorite of fans.

Ingredients:

- 3/4 cup mayonnaise
- 14 oz. bag coleslaw mix
- 3 tablespoons erythritol, confectioners
- 1 1/2 tablespoons lemon juice
- 1 tablespoon apple cider vinegar
- 1 teaspoon dijon mustard
- 1/2 teaspoon celery salt
- 1/2 teaspoon black pepper

Directions:

Whisk the erythritol, mayonnaise, celery salt, black pepper, dijon mustard, lemon juice, and vinegar together in an about a medium bowl. Insert the Mix together well. Change salt and pepper according to taste.

Additional notes:

Refrigerate to allow the flavor to mix for 60 minutes or longer. Mix up until serving.

Nutritional information:

Serving Size: 1/2 cup, Yield: 6 servings

Amount per Serving: Carbohydrates: 10g, Protein: 1g, Calories: 205, Total Fiber: 2g, Net Carbohydrates: 2g, Sugar Alcohols: 6g, Total Fat: 20g

6.2 Buffalo Chicken Soup (Low Carb, Gluten-Free)

Yield: Makes 10 Servings, Cooking Time: 7 hours, Prep Time: 15 minutes, Total Time: 7 hours 15 minutes,

Ingredients:

- 32 oz chicken stock
- 1 lb. chicken breast, cubed
- 1/2 cup buffalo wing sauce
- 2 medium carrots, chopped
- 4 green onions, chopped
- 2 ribs celery, diced
- 1 cup sharp cheddar cheese, shredded
- 2 cloves garlic, minced
- 2/3 cup Parmesan cheese, shredded
- 2 tbsp Italian flat-leaf parsley, chopped (for garnish)
- 1/4 cup blue cheese crumbles, extra to garnish if needed

Instructions:

Slowly heat the cooker on low flame.

Add chicken, buffalo wing sauce, chicken stock, green onion, celery, garlic, and carrots to slow cooker—cover and boil for six hours.

Then add cheddar, cream cheese, and parmesan cheese. Mix until the cheeses are blended in and melted. Cover and simmer for 1 hour.

Before presenting, garnish with crumbles of blue cheese and with parsley.

Nutrition:

Per Serving – Fat: 4g | Calories: 146 | Net Carbs: 3g | Protein: 13g

6.3 Creamy Reuben Soup

Yield: Makes 14 servings Cooking Time: 6 hours Prep Time: 20 minutes, Total Time: 6 hours 20 minutes,

Ingredients:

- 2 ribs celery, diced
- 1 medium onion, diced
- 2 large cloves garlic, minced
- 1 ½ cup Swiss cheese, shredded
- 1 lb. corned beef, chopped
- 3 tbsp butter
- 4 cups beef stock
- 1 tsp sea salt
- 1 cup sauerkraut
- 1 tsp caraway seeds
- 2 cups heavy cream
- ¾ tsp black pepper

Instructions:

Heat up with high setting the slow cooker.

Add celery, onion, butter, and garlic on low, medium heat, to the big sauté pan. Stir in until smooth but also translucent. Shift to your slow cooker.

Add beef stock, corned beef, sauerkraut, caraway seed, sea salt, and the black pepper to the slow cooker. Cover for 4.5 hours and cook on warm.

Add Swiss cheese & heavy cream, and cook for another 1 hour.

Nutrition:

Per Serving –Fat: 18.5g | Calories: 225 | Net Carbs: 4g | Protein: 11.5g

6.4 Keto Bacon Cheeseburger Soup

Yield: 12 servings, Cooking Time: 60 Minutes, Prep Time: 20 Minutes, Total Time: 1 hour 20 minutes,

Ingredients:

- 1 medium tomato, diced (or a 14.5 ounce can dice tomatoes)
- 4 cups beef stock
- 1/3 cup chopped dill pickles
- 2 tablespoons of Worcestershire sauce
- 2 tablespoons Dijon Mustard
- 2 tablespoons chopped fresh flat-leaf parsley
- ½ teaspoon black pepper
- 1 teaspoon sea salt, more to taste
- 1 ½ pound of ground beef
- 4 cloves of garlic, minced
- 1 small onion, diced
- 1 1/2 cups cheddar cheese
- 8 slices bacon, cooked crisp and crumbled
- 1 cup heavy cream

Instructions:

SLOW COOKER SETTING:

In low setting, heat the slow cooker.

Add the beef supply, Worcestershire sauce, onions, dijon, parsley, pickles, black pepper, and sea salt to the slow cooker.

Cook the onions, ground beef, and garlic in a large skillet over medium to high heat until your ground beef is cooked and browned completely and thoroughly. Drain the extra fat and add it to your slow cooker – cover and boil for 6 hours.

Mix in heavy cream and cheddar cheese, and cook 1 extra hour.

Just before eating, whisk in bacon.

STOVETOP INSTRUCTIONS:

Heat the large Dutch oven over medium heat or stockpot. Add the onions, ground beef, and garlic and cook until browned and the ground beef is cooked through.

Then add the stock of beef, tomatoes, pickles, Worcestershire sauce, dijon, parsley, black pepper, and sea salt; Bring to a boil, then rising to medium-low heat and simmer 30 minutes.

Add in the heavy cream and cheddar cheese, reduce heat to medium, regularly cover and whisk, simmer for about 30 minutes.

Just before eating, whisk in bacon.

Nutrition:

Serving Size: 1 cup, Fat: 11g, Calories: 306, Protein: 13g Carbohydrates: 3 net g

6.5 Whole30 Cabbage Roll Soup

Yield: 16 cups Cooking Time: 45 Minutes, Prep Time: 15 Minutes, Total Time: 1 hour,

Ingredients:

- 2 tablespoons olive oil
- 2 tablespoons butter or ghee

- 1 cup diced onion
- 1 1/2 pounds ground beef
- 4 cloves garlic, minced
- 6 cups beef stock
- 1/2-pound ground pork
- 3 teaspoons dried oregano leaves
- 2 teaspoons smoked paprika
- 2 teaspoon of sea salt
- 2 teaspoons garlic powder
- 1 large head cabbage, halved and sliced
- 1 teaspoon black pepper
- 2 teaspoons onion powder
- 1/2 teaspoon dried thyme
- 6 ounce can tomato paste
- (2) 14.5-ounce cans diced tomatoes, drained
- 2 tablespoons chopped fresh flat-leaf parsley
- 3 cups riced cauliflower

Instructions:

Warm the oil and butter in an oven or stockpot on medium flame. Stir in the garlic and onion.

Add your ground pork and beef to the saucepan. Cook until they are brown then wash any extra oil. Add the oregano, cabbage, beef broth, sea salt, riced cauliflower, garlic oil, ointment oil, thyme, paprika, black pepper, onions, parsley, and tomato paste. After boiling point, decrease the heat and simmer them for 30 to 45 minutes.

Nutrition:

Serving Size: 1 cup, Fat: 12.9g, Calories: 200, Fiber: 4g, Carbohydrates: 10.5 net grams, Protein: 12.1g

6.6 Low Carb Slow Cooker Kickin' Chili

Cooking Time: 8 hours, Prep Time: 30 minutes, Total Time: 8 hours 30 minutes

Ingredients:

- 1 medium red onion, chopped and divided
- 2 1/2 pounds ground beef
- 5 cloves garlic, minced
- 1/4 cup pickled jalapeno slices
- 3 large ribs of celery, diced
- 6 ounce can tomato paste
- 14.5 ounce can stew tomatoes
- 14.5 ounce can tomato and green chilies
- 2 tablespoons Worcestershire sauce or Coconut Aminos
- 2 tablespoons cumin, mounded
- 4 tablespoons chili powder
- 2 teaspoons sea salt
- 1 bay leaf
- 1 teaspoon onion powder
- 1 teaspoon garlic powder
- 1 teaspoon oregano
- 1/2 teaspoon cayenne
- 1 teaspoon black pepper

Instructions:

In low setting, heat the slow cooker.

Put ground beef in a wide skillet on medium-high heat, half the onions, 2 Tablespoons, Seasoned garlic, salt, and pepper. Drain extra grease from the saucepan once your beef gives brown color.

Shift ground beef to slow cooker. Add the remaining garlic, onions, celery, tomato paste, jalapenos, tomatoes and, stewed tomatoes (along with liquid), chilies (along with liquid) chili powder, Worcestershire sauce, cumin, cayenne, salt, garlic powder, oregano, onion powder, bay leaf, and black pepper.

Remove until all the ingredients combine well — Cook for 6-8 hours at medium.

Nutrition:

Per Serving: 1 Cup | Fat: 5g | Calories: 137 | Net Carbs: 4.7g | Protein: 16g

6.7 Low Carb Cauliflower and Broccoli Cheese Soup

Yield: Makes 16 servings Cooking Time: 6 hours, Prep Time: 20 minutes, Total Time: 6 hours 20 minutes,

Ingredients:

- 1 medium onion, chopped
- 2 tbsp butter
- 5 cloves garlic, minced
- 1 medium cauliflower
- Sea salt and black pepper, to taste
- 1 1/2 lbs. broccoli, cut into small florets
- 4 cups chicken stock
- 1 leek, cleaned and trimmed
- 2 cups heavy cream
- 2 cups Parmesan cheese, grated
- 4 cups sharp cheddar cheese, shredded

Instructions:

Heat over medium heat a big, sauté pan. Add butter, garlic, onion, black pepper, and marine salt to the saucepan. Sauté the onions until onions are caramelized and nice for about twenty Minutes. Heat up on high setting slow cooker. Add broccoli, caramelized onions, leek, heavy cream, chicken stock, and a small amount of black pepper and sea salt.

Blend both materials. Cover for 5-6 hours, and cook on high.

The vegetables should be soft and tender after 5–6 hours. Mash-up the vegetables using the potato masher. Alternatively, this can be done using your immersion blender.

Mix in Parmesan and cheddar cheeses, add salt and pepper, and allow 1 extra hour to cook.

Nutrition:

Per Serving – Fat: 18g | Calories: 235| Net Carbs: 5g | Protein: 13g

Serving Size: 1 Cup, Fat: 18g, Calories: 235.

6.8 Keto Smoked Sausage Cheddar Beer Soup

Yield: 14 servings Cooking Time: 6 Hours, Prep Time: 30 Minutes, Total Time: 6 hours 30 minutes.

Ingredients:

- 4 cups beef stock
- 14 ounces beef smoked sausage, sliced and halved
- A 12-ounce bottle of gluten-free beer (optional – can substitute extra beef stock or even non-alcoholic beer)
- 1 cup chopped celery
- 1 cup chopped carrots
- 1 small onion, diced
- 2 cups shredded sharp cheddar cheese
- 1 teaspoon red pepper flakes

- 4 cloves garlic, minced
- 1 teaspoon sea salt, more to taste
- 1 cup heavy cream
- 1/2 teaspoon black pepper
- 8 ounces cream cheese

Instructions:

At high setting, heat your slow cooker.

Add beef stock, sausage, carrot, beer, celery, onion, carrot, garlic, pepper, and sea salt to your slow cooker — Cook 4 hours on high.

Add the cheddar cheese, heavy cheese, and cream cheese. Stir until cream cheese clumps do not exist anymore. Use a whisk in that process — Cook for another 2 hours.

Nutrition:

Serving Size: 1 cup, Fat: 17g, Calories: 244, Fiber: 5g Carbohydrates: 4 net grams,

6.9 Low Carb Boneless Buffalo wings

Yield: Makes 4 servings Cooking Time: 30 minutes, Prep Time: 30 minutes, Total Time: 1 hour,

Ingredients:

- 1 1/2 cups crushed pork rinds
- Oil for frying
- 1-pound boneless chicken breast
- 1/2 cup grated Parmesan cheese
- 3/4 cup buffalo wing sauce
- 1/2 teaspoon garlic powder
- 2 tablespoons butter

Instructions:

Cut the extra fat off the chicken breast and cut into the large chunks.

Combine Parmesan cheese, garlic powder, and pork rinds, and pulse in the food processor until the ingredients are all well mixed and relatively fine. Press the paste onto a thin film onto a tray.

Steam a centimeter of oil on medium to high temperature. You can use the nonstick wok for deep frying on the stovetop. The high sides minimize splattering and render a cinch safe.

Press chicken pieces tightly into your breading mixture, wrapping all sides (To do so, it will make the breading attach to the chicken even more than just stirring them in breading mixture).

As the oil is hot, drop the breaded chicken in the oil. By using tongs, you can flip the pieces of chicken a few times till both sides are crispy and golden brown – approximately 3 minutes each.

After having removed chicken from the oil, allow it to cool to soak excess grease on a paper towel. It would also include an opportunity for the breading to crisp up, and it remains on.

Melt your butter and then mix in sauce with the buffalo wing. Toss the chicken lightly into the sauce.

Nutrition:

Per Serving –Fat: 15g | Calories: 350 | Net Carbs: 0.5g | Protein: 40g

6.10 Pickled Red Onions

It is a perfect mixture of sweet, salty, and sour. You'll enjoy using those onions on anything that can be your early pancakes, to the lunchtime bowl, to top of your dinner steak.

Yield: 20 Servings Cooking Time: 5 Minutes, Prep Time: 15 Minutes, Total Time: 20 minutes,

Ingredients:

- 1 cup apple cider vinegar
- 2 tablespoons granular monk fruit or erythritol granular
- 1 cup red wine vinegar
- Pinch of red pepper flakes
- 1 teaspoon of sea salt
- 6 cloves garlic, peeled and halved
- 2 medium red onions, thinly sliced
- 1 teaspoon dried oregano leaves

Instructions:

Combine the apple cider vinegar, erythritol, red wine vinegar, and salt in a saucepan on medium heat. Bring it to a light boil, mixing until the salt and erythritol are dissolved.

In a thirty-two-ounce Mason jar, placed the oregano, garlic, onions, and the red pepper flakes.

In the red pepper flakes and oregano, pour liquid on the top, submerge the onions and blend.

Let the container stay on your counter for one hour, then cap and cool off.

Keep in the fridge for a period of 2 months. You should consume them after two hours, so the longer they're in the fridge they'll get only better and better.

Nutrition:

Serving Size: 5-6 slices, Fat: 0, Calories: 10, Carbohydrates: 1.5g, Protein: 0.2g, Fiber: 0.2g

6.11 Pickled Jalapeños

Yield: 20 servings Cooking Time: 10 minutes, Prep Time: 10 minutes, Total Time: 20 minutes,

Ingredients:

- 3 cloves garlic, peeled and halved
- 10 jalapeños
- 2 tablespoons granular erythritol
- 1 teaspoon yellow mustard seed
- 1 cup white vinegar
- 1/2 teaspoon dried oregano
- 1 cup of water
- 1 teaspoon of sea salt

Instructions:

Cut the jalapeños from the stems and cut them into 1/4-inch circles.

Place sliced jalapeños and mustard seed, garlic, and oregano in a thirty-two-ounce mason jar.

Combine the water, erythritol, vinegar, and salt in a saucepan on medium heat. Boil it lightly and then stir until the salt and erythritol are dissolved.

Pour the liquid on the top, submerge the jalapeños and mix in oregano.

Let the container stay on your counter for one hour, then cap and cool off.

Keep in the fridge for a period of 2 months. You might consume them after 2 days, so the longer they're in the freezer, they'll only get better and better.

Nutrition:

Net carbohydrates per serving=0.4g

Serving Size: 1 serving, Fat: 0.1g, Calories: 3, Carbohydrates: 0.7g, Protein: 0.1g, Fiber: 0.2g

6.12 Creamy Chive Blue Cheese Dressing

Total Time: 5 minutes, Prep Time: 5 minutes, Yield: 2 1/2 cups

Ingredients:

- 1/2 cup sour cream
- 1 cup mayonnaise
- 1 tablespoon fresh lemon juice
- 1 teaspoon garlic powder
- 1 teaspoon Worcestershire sauce
- 1/2 teaspoon sea salt
- 3/4 cup crumbled blue cheese
- 1/2 teaspoon black pepper
- 1/4 cup chopped fresh chives

Instructions:

Add the ingredients in a pot and then blend well until mixed.

Nutrition:

Serving Size: 2 tbsp, Fat: 12g, Calories: 106, Protein: 1g Carbohydrates: 1g,

6.13 Low Carb Taco Seasoning

It is a fast and simple seasoning on Low Carb Taco. You can skip ingredients and produce your own in store-bought taco seasoning.

Yield: 1 batch Cook Time: 0 minutes, Prep Time: 5 minutes, Total Time: 5 minutes,

Ingredients:

- 2 tablespoons cumin
- ½ teaspoon black pepper

- 2 tablespoons chili powder
- 2 teaspoons onion powder
- 2 teaspoons celery salt
- 2 teaspoons garlic powder
- ½ teaspoon cayenne pepper
- ½ teaspoon of sea salt

Instructions:

Mix all the ingredients in a jar.

Nutrition:

Serving Size=1 batch, Fat: 5g, Calories: 151, Protein: 7g, Carbohydrates: 15g,

6.14 Paleo 2 Minute Avocado Oil Mayo (Whole30)

Yield: 15 tbsp

Ingredients:

- 1 cup avocado oil
- 2 teaspoons lemon juice
- 1/2 teaspoon dry mustard powder
- 1 large egg
- 1/2 teaspoon sea salt

Instructions:

Add lemon juice first to a big, largemouth mason's jar, then egg, seasonings, and finally oil. Let all ingredients sit for approximately 20 seconds.

Place your immersion blender into the mason's jar completely. Turn it at high speed, and leave for about twenty seconds at the bottom of your jar. The mayo will begin setting up and filling the jar right away.

Slowly pull your immersion blender to the top of the pot, without getting blades out of mayonnaise, until your mayonnaise is placed nearly all the way. Then, push it back slowly towards the bottom of the jar. Repeat the phase a few times till all of your ingredients are very well integrated.

If you want, taste and add some more salt.

Nutrition:

Serving Size=1 tbsp, Sodium: 82mg, Calories: 134, Fat: 14.9g, Carbohydrates: 0.1g, Saturated Fat: 1.8g, Protein: 0.4g

6.15 Muffuletta Olive Salad

Total Time: Ten minutes, Prep Time: 10 minutes, Yield: 20 Servings

Ingredients:

- 1 cup of green olives
- 1 1/2 cups giardiniera pickled vegetables
- 1 cup Kalamata olives
- 1/3 cup red wine vinegar
- 1/2 cup pepperoncini
- 1/4 cup roasted red peppers
- 4 large cloves garlic
- 1/2 cup capers
- 1/4 cup olive oil
- 1 teaspoon dried oregano leaves
- 1/2 teaspoon black pepper
- 1 teaspoon dried basil

Instructions:

Mix the giardiniera, kalamata olives, green olives, olive oil, pepperoncini, roasted red peppers, red vinegar, and garlic in your food processor. Pulse until roughly all of your ingredients are chopped.

Pulse until it is incorporated in the black pepper, basil, and oregano.

Stir capers in. Cover and cool for a total of one hour before serving

Nutrition:

2g net carbohydrates per serving

Serving Size=1/4 Cup, Fat: 5g, Calories: 56, Carbohydrates: 2g

6.16 Avocado Ranch Dressing (Low Carbohydrates and Gluten-Free)

Total Time=10 minutes, Prep Time=10 minutes, Yield=twelve Servings

Ingredients:

- ½ cup mayonnaise
- 1/2 large avocado, pitted and peeled
- ½ cup of sour cream
- 1/8 tablespoon black pepper
- 1 tablespoon fresh parsley and chopped
- 1 clove garlic that is minced
- ¼ tsp sea salt
- 1 tbsp fresh chives that are chopped
- 1 tsp fresh dill, chopped
- 2 tablespoon apple cider vinegar
- ½ tablespoon onion powder

Directions:

Slush the avocado with a fork in a large mixing bowl. Add sour cream, mayonnaise, garlic, chives, parsley, and vinegar with apple cider, onion powder, dill, black pepper, and sea salt to avocado. Mix all the ingredients until properly incorporated. Refrigerate for a total of 1 hour before eating.

Nutrition:

Per Serving –Fat: 10g | Net Carbohydrates: 1g | Calories: 100 | Protein:7g

Serving Size=two tablespoon

6.17 Keto Russian Dressing

Total Time: 5 minutes Prep Time: 5 minutes Yield: 8 servings

Ingredients:

- ½ cup reduced sugar ketchup
- 1 cup mayonnaise
- 1 teaspoon chopped fresh dill
- 2 tablespoons spicy brown mustard
- 1 tablespoon chopped fresh parsley
- 1 tablespoon Worcestershire sauce
- 1 tablespoon chopped fresh chives

Instructions:

Combine ketchup, mayonnaise, mustard, dill, chives, Worcestershire sauce, and parsley in the large mixing bowl. Mix all ingredients until they are properly incorporated.

Nutrition:

Serving Size=1/4 cup, Fat: 20g, Calories: 190, Carbohydrates: 1.5g, Protein: 0g, Fiber: 0g,

6.18 Dairy-Free Keto Ranch Dressing

Yield=12 servings

Ingredients:

- 1/4 cup water
- 1 cup mayonnaise
- 1/2 teaspoon black pepper
- 2 teaspoons chopped fresh chives
- 1 teaspoon Dijon mustard

- 1 teaspoon chopped fresh dill weed
- 1 teaspoon garlic powder
- 1 teaspoon chopped fresh flat-leaf parsley
- 1/2 teaspoon onion powder
- 1/2 teaspoon sea salt

Instructions:

Combine all the ingredients in the Mason jar, then cap, and then combine to shake. Alternatively, in the mixing bowl, together, you can mix all the ingredients and whisk till it's incorporated.

Nutrition:

Serving Size=2 tbsp., Fat: 13g, Calories: 122, Fiber: 0g, Carbohydrates: .3g, Protein: 0g

6.19 Whole30 Cabbage Roll Soup

Yield: 16 cups Cook Time: 45 Minutes, Prep Time: 15 Minutes, Total Time: 1 hour,

Ingredients:

- 2 tablespoons olive oil
- 2 tablespoons butter or ghee
- 1 cup diced onion
- 1 1/2 pounds ground beef
- 4 cloves garlic, minced
- 1/2-pound ground pork
- 3 teaspoons dried oregano leaves
- 6 cups beef stock
- 2 teaspoon of sea salt
- 2 teaspoons garlic powder
- 1 large head cabbage, halved and sliced
- 2 teaspoons smoked paprika
- 2 teaspoons onion powder
- 1/2 teaspoon dried thyme

- 1 teaspoon black pepper
- 6 ounce can tomato paste
- (2) 14.5-ounce cans diced tomatoes, drained
- 2 tablespoons chopped fresh flat-leaf parsley
- 3 cups riced cauliflower

Instructions:

Warm butter and olive oil in a big Dutch oven or stockpot on medium heat. Stir in the ginger and onion. Cook until translucent onion, then fragrant with garlic.

Add the pork and ground beef to the saucepan. Cook them until browned, and drain any grease in excess. Add oregano, beef broth, sea salt, garlic oil, paprika, ointment oil, black pepper, cabbage, thyme, onions, parsley, tomato paste, and the riced cauliflower. Bring to a boil, then rising to low heat and then simmer for 30 to 45 minutes.

Nutrition:

6.5g net carbohydrates per serving

Serving Size=1 cup, Fat: 12.9g, Calories: 200, Carbohydrates: 10.5 net grams, Protein: 12.1g Fiber: 4g.

6.20 Ketogenic Breakfast Smoothie

Keto Summit

Ingredients:

- Spinach
- Coconut milk
- Greens powder
- Almonds
- Brazil nuts
- Whey protein
- Psyllium seeds (or psyllium husks)
- Potato starch

This great green smoothie recipe uses both new spinach and Incredible Grass greens material. Drop for its selenium in some brazil nuts and some almonds for a nutty taste, and you have a balanced, safe, and tasty keto breakfast smoothie.

6.21 Keto Spinach Avocado Green Smoothie

Keto Summit

Ingredients:

- Coconut milk (unsweetened –from refrigerated cartons, not cans)
- Avocado
- Spinach (or other leafy greens)
- Vanilla extract
- Sweetener

Not all smoothies are made equal, but you can safely bet that this green smoothie keto spinach avocado is tasty as well as nutritious!

6.22 Keto Lemon Ginger Green Juice Shots

Keto Summit

Ingredients:

- Kale
- Celery stalks
- Lemon juice
- Generous handful of mint leaves
- Fresh Ginger
- Erythritol

Seek some shots of green juice from Keto lemon ginger if you're searching for a lift.

6.23 Green Keto Smoothie with Avocado and Mint

Low Carb Yum

Ingredients:

- Coconut milk
- Almond milk
- Avocado
- Sweetener
- Mint
- Cilantro
- Lime
- Vanilla
- Ice

Don't get bored with keto green smoothies! There are a ton of variations, and this green keto smoothie recipe is refreshing and packed with nutrients. Don't omit the avocado in this drink -it makes the smoothie thicker and creamier.

6.24 Chocolate Green Smoothie

Ditch the Carbs

Ingredients:

- Coconut cream
- Frozen berries of choice
- Spinach
- Cocoa powder
- Granulated sweetener of choice.

Enjoy this simple keto smoothie recipe with a fruity but still chocolaty cocktail. And when you're at it for additional protein, you may as well mix in some spinach!

6.25 Keto Avocado Smoothie

Ingredients:

- Vanilla extract
- Avocado
- Coconut milk
- Ice
- Stevia, or erythritol.

Do not place the ketosis at risk by making a 'good' smoothie packed with sugar and carbohydrates. This velvety avocado smoothie is great for your diet and is completely ketogenic.

6.26 Keto Avocado Apple Coconut Smoothie

Ingredients:

- Apple
- Coconut milk (unsweetened, from a carton)
- Avocado
- Lime juice
- MCT oil
- Collagen powder
- Unsweetened shredded coconut.

Want a Keto smoothie made of good fats and tons of flavors? Then give this avocado smoothie a try -it's flavored with delicious apples and coconut!

6.27 Keto Blueberry Ginger Smoothie

Ingredients:

- Coconut yogurt
- Blueberries
- Coconut milk
- Ginger

- Apple
- MCT oil
- Collagen powder
- Stevia

Sometimes, MCT oil is deemed awesome to raise ketone rates. So why not incorporate Keto smoothies and shakes into your morning! Definitely, this blueberry treat can inspire you to add some good fat to your morning coffee.

6.28 Low Carb Strawberry Crunch Smoothie

Ingredients:

- Strawberries
- Cinnamon
- Unsweetened vanilla almond milk
- Almonds
- Chia seeds (optional)

If you're hunting for a low-carb fruity smoothie, therefore this one is for you. This smoothie will give you the pleasure you are searching for, with soft, sweet strawberry and a touch of spicy cinnamon.

6.29 "Sleep In" Smoothie

Ingredients:

- Water or Coconut milk or almond milk
- Egg
- Fruit (mix of berries)
- Avocado
- Fresh spinach

The idea for this ketogenic smoothie recipe is fantastic - it's a super simple but yet nice-tasting cocktail you might also create when you roll out of bed!

6.30 Strawberry Coconut Smoothie

Ingredients:

- Strawberries
- Nut Milk
- Coconut manna
- Chia seed
- Shredded coconut (optional)

Coconut and strawberries are an ideal mix for a delicious and sweet treat. This smoothie is not just tasty, with only five basic ingredients, but also a very fast and convenient recipe to produce. Only take in your supplies and put them together.

6.31 Coconut Cherry Vanilla Smoothie

Ingredients:

- Water
- Vanilla powder
- Coconut milk
- Ground sea salt
- Frozen organic sweet cherries
- Ice cubes

What could taste better than Vanilla and cherries? A keto smoothie and coconut milk produced from both! Without being too sweet, this tasty treat will certainly curb the desire for sweets.

6.32 Blueberry Power Shake

Ingredients:

- Blueberries or strawberries
- Stevia
- Coconut milk
- Vanilla extract

- Virgin coconut oil (optional but recommended)
- Gelatin (optional but recommended)
- Ice cubes

This formula for power shake is super simple to create and has just a few ingredients, making it a perfect cocktail for anyone in a rush. This has a fantastic flavor while ensuring that you get a good dose of fats every day.

6.33 Coconut Milk Strawberry Smoothie

Ingredients:

- Unsweetened coconut milk
- Frozen strawberries
- Almond butter
- Stevia

Keto smoothie recipes can be really simple -like this one. This is packed with good fats and wonderful aromas of strawberry. Then what you have to do is pour all in and mix it all together.

6.34 Low Carb Strawberry Smoothie

Ingredients:

- Frozen strawberries
- Unsweetened Almond milk
- Avocado
- Erythritol

Frozen berries are fantastic to add to your Keto smoothie recipes. You save the hassle of having to add in extra ice cubes to chill your drink.

Conclusion

For many people, a keto diet can be a healthy choice, but the ratio of fat, carbs, and protein required can vary from person to person.

If you are diabetic, discuss the diet with your doctor before beginning, as it will likely involve medication adjustments and increased blood sugar control.

On High blood pressure medication? Consult with your doctor before you continue a keto diet again.

If you are breastfeeding, don't continue a keto diet.

Be aware that restricting carbs will, among other possibilities, make you feel irritable, hungry, and tired. That, however, may be a temporary effect.

Do remember your diet should be healthy, so you get all the vitamins and minerals you need. Enough fiber is also essential.

Ketosis happens when the body starts extracting energy from stored fat rather than glucose.

Several studies have demonstrated the strong effects of a low carb diet, or keto, on weight loss. This diet can be hard to maintain, however, and can cause health problems in people with certain conditions, such as type 1 diabetes.

Most people can safely seek out the keto diet. Nonetheless, it is best to talk to a dietitian or doctor about any significant changes to the diet. This is basically the case for those with disabilities underlying it.

A successful treatment for people with drug-resistant epilepsy could be the keto diet.

While the diet can be ideal for people of any age, children, and people over the age of 50, and infants may enjoy the greatest benefits as they can easily adhere to the diet.

Adolescents and adults, such as the modified Atkins diet or the low-glycemic index diet, can do better on a modified keto diet.

A health care provider should track closely; whoever is using a keto diet as a medication.

A doctor and dietitian are able to monitor the progress of a person, prescribe medications, and test for adverse effects.

The body processes fat differently from that it processes protein differently from that of carbohydrates. The Carbohydrate response to insulin is very strong. The protein response to insulin is moderate, and the fast response to the insulin is very small. Insulin is the hormone that produces fat / conserves fat. Eat all the eggs, poultry, fish, birds you want, satiate with the fat on, and then eat any vegetable that grows on the ground if you want to lose weight. Stop pressed synthetic seed oils in favor of butter and coconut oil. You can be a sugar burner or a fat burner, but you can't be both.

Printed in Great Britain
by Amazon

23105894R00079